THE
QUEEN

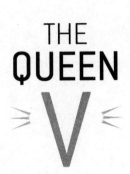

THE
QUEEN

V

EVERYTHING YOU NEED
TO KNOW ABOUT INTIMACY,
SEX, AND **DOWN THERE**
HEALTHCARE

Dr. Jackie Walters

Andy Cohen Books
Henry Holt and Company
New York

Andy Cohen Books
Henry Holt and Company
Publishers since 1866
120 Broadway
New York, New York 10271
www.henryholt.com

Andy Cohen Books® and ★® are registered trademarks of
Macmillan Publishing Group, LLC.
Andy Cohen logo caricature by Robert Risko

Library of Congress Cataloging-in-Publication Data is available
ISBN: 9781250209184

Our books may be purchased in bulk for promotional, educational, or business use. Please
contact your local bookseller or the Macmillan Corporate and Premium Sales Department at
(800) 221-7945, extension 5442, or by email at MacmillanSpecialMarkets@macmillan.com.

First Edition 2020

Illustrations by Laura Hartman Maestro

Designed by Susan Walsh

Printed in the United States of America

1 3 5 7 9 10 8 6 4 2

In the past, people were born royal. Nowadays, royalty comes from what you do.

—Gianni Versace

To Queen Vs everywhere. All hail each and every royal one!

CONTENTS

Preface

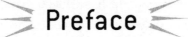

What's powerful enough to make grown men cry and persuasive enough to end a mythological war? What has more elasticity than most rubber bands and more forgiveness than Mother Teresa? This breathtakingly beautiful thing I'm talking about can soothe the greatest pain and inspire the greatest pleasure.

She has been called by many names, but let's use her proper one: your *vagina*.

Now for a tougher question: When was the last time you actually looked at her? Ask yourself if you could identify her in a lineup (an incredibly unlikely lineup, but you see where I'm going). My point is that we tend to ignore that infinitely strong, influential, and exquisite organ between our legs until something goes wrong. And even then, we don't always go to the right sources, nor do we ask the right questions at the right time. Believe me, I know, because I've been there too.

At the age of ten, I saw my cousins hiding mysterious pads in the bathroom. I was confused and a bit traumatized. What was going on? What *were* those things?

When my time came, my momma only offered up the basics of what was necessary for me to know, and I started a ritual of wrapping my pads up and tucking them way at the bottom of the garbage can where no one would accidentally see them. Out of sight, out of mind, I hoped. Just like the yellow box of Massengill hidden in my mother's closet and the mysterious red hot-water bottle with a tube sticking out that hung on the back of her bathroom door. There was never any mention of sex or what a period could mean beyond a monthly annoyance. I was so ignorant and ashamed of my own femininity and sexuality for years. And I suspect today there are still moms who don't talk to their daughters about sexuality. So we grow up in silence and walk into relationships and marriages so intimately blind that we end up sexually cosigning on things that aren't right for *us*.

But as I grew up, I found I was passionate about health and taking care of women, which led me to study medicine and become a board-certified obstetrician and gynecologist with my own practice in Atlanta. It took me years to unlearn much of what I saw and what I thought in my adolescence so I could learn what I needed to know to become a confident woman—and help other women become confident too.

There's so much that all us women need to know about intimacy, our bodies, and our sexuality. Not everyone's having the twenty-first-century conversations about sex that I wish they were. That changes today—with this book.

By the time you finish reading this book, you'll be able to communicate with your doctor, your partner, and your girlfriends in ways you never thought possible. You'll deepen intimacy in your relationships, you'll be empowered to handle sexual health problems with less fear, and you'll get a heads-up on what everyone else is doing (but not necessarily talking about) in case you want to join them.

This book is full of stories about patients I've encountered over the decades. Their experiences will help you see that your own story isn't unusual and get an idea of how other women have dealt with similar issues and concerns. I do take doctor-patient confidentiality extremely seriously, so I haven't included anyone's name and I've changed identifying details about them.

You should know this book is for everyone who owns or loves a vagina. In my practice I see heterosexual women, lesbian women, bisexual women, asexual women, and trans people. I realize that not all women have vaginas and that not everyone with a vagina thinks of themselves as a woman. I also get tons of questions from men. So if you're curious about how to hail a Queen V (or vagina), I'm talking to you in these pages. In celebration of our Queen Vs, I use a lot of slang terms when I reference her. Embrace what fits and let go of what doesn't. It's not my intent to exclude anyone who uses different language than I do or identifies in a different way. My goal is to educate you about sexual health, empower you—and hopefully give you some laughs, surprises, and reassurance along the way.

Some people want to save the trees. I'm here to save the vaginas. And if you've got one, I'm starting with yours.

How to Read This Book

Just like a shirtless hunk walking past you on the beach, you can read this book from top to bottom and front to back. However, I do encourage you to start with the introduction, where you'll meet your VP—your Vaginal Personality. In my practice, I have found that there are five different types of women when it comes to their relationship to their vagina, and identifying yours will go a long way to understanding your physical and sexual self.

It has taken me almost two decades of wearing a white coat and putting my arms around women, listening to them, examining them, saving their lives, and consoling them, to pull the golden rules in this book together. To keep it (relatively) simple, I organized the book into twelve principles I want all women to follow when it comes to their sexual health. And if you follow them, I guarantee they'll change your sexual life.

I've filled this book with patient anecdotes from my years of practice, and if a specific chapter doesn't apply to an issue you're having, I think you'll still want to read up. By pulling back the exam curtain on everything from sex-enhancing surgery to mysterious periods, what you learn in these pages could help your sister, your mother, your best friend, or yourself. If you need help in a specific area, just scroll through the table of contents or hit the index in the back to find what you're looking for. I've tried to make this book as comprehensive as possible when it comes to women's sexual health, so you'll see everything from intimacy to infertility in these pages.

And, finally, I ask that you don't just read in silence—please share what you've learned with your circle so we all become more knowledgeable and open when it comes to our vaginas and our health.

Introduction

I want to let you in on a secret. It's something I wish someone had told me decades ago.

Since getting my MD, as a board-certified OB-GYN in Atlanta I've sat down with thousands of women at all stages of their lives. Celebrities you're used to seeing onstage, I'm used to seeing in the stirrups. But you don't have to have a high profile to book an appointment with me. Regular folks who shop in Target (just like I do) walk through the door of my private practice.

And while each and every woman I ask to put on a paper gown is absolutely unique, I have noticed some similarities among them. And it's time I told everyone about those similarities.

The secret is that you, my dear, have a VP—and I'm about to introduce you to her.

WHAT EXACTLY IS A VP?

It's your Vaginal Personality, and in my decades of practice, I've found there are five types. I've named them for the sake of clarity—and I think these names are pretty accurate—the Virgin Mary, the Sanctified Snatch, the Mary Jane, the Coochie-Chondriac, and the Notorious V.A.G.

Your VP can dictate everything from how soon you call me about a problem you're having down there to how soon you take a man home with you after you meet him. Your VP often indicates how much detail you offer when you're sharing your sexual history with me at an appointment and how much detail you offer your sexual partner about how to bring you to climax. It's how introverted or extroverted you are. How outspoken or quiet you are. It's how adventurous or reserved you are. It's your sexual compass, sensual temperament, and the guardian of your vaginal health all rolled into one.

Intimate knowledge of your VP is absolutely essential for every woman. Knowing your VP and taking charge of your relationship to your own vagina will change your life—your VP has the power to prevent you from spending all weekend freaking out about a "strange" discharge, and it can keep you from accidentally getting pregnant. Embracing your VP can even take your sex life from ho-hum to, well, hotter than the ATL.

But women rarely think about their relationships to their own sexual health and their VPs—and don't get me started on their actual vaginas. Often, we only consider them when it's time for our annual appointment or when there's a problem in our relationship, like sexual incompatibility. Be honest. You've probably spent more time thinking about what to watch on Netflix this week than about your vagina—unless you have a problem going on. And that's fair, considering you probably haven't heard of a VP until this very moment. But this moment is about to change everything.

HOW I FOUND MY VP

My first VP (that's right, they can change over time!) was definitely dictated by my upbringing, which made me entirely, undeniably, and unapologetically a "Sanctified Snatch" (or an SS, for shorthand). You probably know someone just like I was: prim and proper, kindhearted, churchgoing, and oh-so-classy. The kind of girl who is definitely down to, ahem, make love but also "cleans up" right after sex.

I grew up very sheltered, and my parents, who were both schoolteachers, taught me to uphold a certain image of propriety. I needed to dress a certain way (i.e., conservatively: no boobs hanging out, no short skirts, and definitely no bare legs. That's what stockings were for). I had to speak properly (no cursing and you better enunciate each word). And I certainly was expected to refrain from sex before marriage.

The story was the same for the circle of women that I tended to hang out with. As an SS, it would've been heresy to hang out with a Notorious V.A.G., for example. (If the name doesn't give it away, all you need to know is that she's your carefree, life-of-the-party type. I like *having fun*. Notorious V.A.G.s like *being the fun*.) Back then, hanging with a Notorious V.A.G. would've spelled trouble. Not much has changed, but these days I do think that trouble (in moderation) can be fun.

Once I got to college, things started to change because I was exposed to so many different types of friends: girls who would show up at a boy's door wearing nothing under a trench coat, frat boys who serenade you outside your window by singing "I'm going to hit you with sperm until you squirm!" (No joke, that actually happened.) But the real turn came when I met my now-husband, Curtis. He respected me as the Sanctified Snatch I was, but after marriage, he got bored—so we got more adventurous. And this Sanctified Snatch turned into more of a Mary Jane—by kicking my sexy up a notch. You'll learn more about that VP later.

LET'S TALK ABOUT SEX . . . AND YOUR VP

Break out your pencil because it's time for a pop quiz. One of the best ways to figure out your VP (besides booking an appointment with me) is by taking this multiple-choice test that I designed. The most important thing to remember about this quiz is to be *honest*. Don't give the answer that you wish were true or that was true for you five years ago. You've got to pick the answer that reflects where you are right here and right now in your life. Don't judge your answers (again, that might make you change them). And don't take this quiz with your best friend (see previous comment about tweaking your answers). If you truly want to understand yourself, then cast off embarrassment and embrace who you are with these twenty questions. Add up the point values that correspond to your answer for each question and see where you land in the end.

THE QUIZ: WHAT'S YOUR VAGINAL PERSONALITY?

1. When you pick up your phone to send your partner a sexy message, you:
   a) Put it back down again. That's waaaaay too bold. (+0)
   b) Send a text message saying you can't wait to see him or her again—and *maybe* use the eggplant or peach emoji (+1)
   c) Send a text message—definitely using the eggplant, peach, pointing finger, and splashing sweat emojis (+2)
   d) Hint at what they can expect this evening in a suggestive voicemail (+3)
   e) Pose for a scantily clad Snapchat pic (+4)

2. It's annual appointment time! When your gynecologist walks in the room to examine you, you're usually:
   a) Wearing nothing at all (+4)
   b) Wearing the paper gown (+2)
   c) Wearing the paper gown, your coat, socks, and a nervous smile (+2)
   d) Was I supposed to get undressed? (+1)

3. Your favorite sexual position is:
   a) Missionary (+0)
   b) Spooning or doggie style (+1)
   c) Reverse cowgirl (+2)
   d) The bridge (+3)

4. When you're in a relationship—and you're in the mood—how frequently do you initiate sex with your partner?
   a) Always; I'm a take-charge kind of woman (+4)
   b) Often; why should I sit back and wait for the fun to start? (+3)
   c) Sometimes a girl's gotta do what a girl's gotta do (+2)
   d) Never. I'm a bit shy, and I prefer my partner to take the lead. (+1)

5. Ooh-ooh-ooh! Your partner just tried a new move in bed and you love it. How do you let them know?

    a) I don't need to let them know; they'll figure it out (+0)

    b) I squirm or smile. Body language does the trick (+1)

    c) I moan so they get the picture (+2)

    d) I flat-out tell them how amazing it feels (+3)

6. How honest are you with your gynecologist about your sexual history?

    a) I tell them everything—including a few freaky sexcapades they haven't even asked about (+4)

    b) I'm holding back a little. I've got a few secrets I'm too embarrassed to share. (+3)

    c) I answer every question in detail (+2)

    d) Some things are best left between me and God (+4)

7. Real talk: Would you ever have sex with someone on the first date?

    a) Definitely not. I'd have to get to know them first (+0)

    b) Unlikely, but I never say never (+1)

    c) Maybe. Depends on how fine they are (+2)

    d) Absolutely. If sparks are flying, why wait? (+3)

8. Most of what you know about sex you learned from:

    a) Your sexual partners (+1)

    b) A book, like this one (+1)

    c) The internet (+1)

    d) A family member (+1)

    e) Honestly, I feel like I have a lot to learn (+0)

9. When you're having sex with a partner, you *usually* like the lights:

    a) Off (+0)

    b) On (+1)

10. How many times a year do you visit your OB-GYN—assuming you don't have a chronic problem?

    a) 5+ (+2)

    b) 2–4 (+1)

    c) 0–1 (+0)

11. If you're excited to get it on *outside* the bedroom, you're likely:

    a) Having a dream. You never have sex outside the bedroom (+0)

    b) In the living room because you just didn't make it to the bedroom (+1)

    c) Spicing things up with shower sex or "cooking up" a good time in the kitchen (+2)

    d) Taking it outdoors on your balcony or in a parked car (+3)

12. When you close your eyes to give your Queen V a surprise, which sexual fantasy are you most likely to think about?

    a) Whip out the whips and chains. You're down for a little bondage or a threesome to kick off a hot weekend. (+4)

    b) Pull on the maid's outfit; it's time for some role-playing with a demanding hotel guest (+4)

    c) Your ex ran through the rain to knock on your door and tell you they're sorry. And they want another chance. Starting tonight. (+2)

    d) That person you've had your eye on for a while? They're finally bringing you roses, chocolate, and a night you'll never forget. (+1)

13. How often do you watch pornography?

    a) Never (+0)

    b) Okay, I'll be honest. Once in a while. (+1)

    c) Whenever's clever. Anytime I'm in the mood. (+2)

    d) Watch it? I should be in it. (+3)

14. How close are you with your gynecologist?

    a) We chat like friends, but I don't see her that often (+4)

    b) It's pretty straightforward doctor-patient. I got a hug once. (+3)

    c) BFFs. She's in my favorites section on my phone. (+2)

    d) I have to google her name and address sometimes because I forget it (+1)

    e) Wait, people are close with their down there doctor? (+0)

15. Do you have to be in love with someone before you have sex with them?

    a) Of course! That's why they call it "making love." (+0)

    b) I mean, that would be *nice* but it isn't *necessary* (+1)

    c) That's cute. You've got jokes. (+2)

16. In your most recent relationship, your partner is/was:

    a) A bit of a train wreck who did you wrong. In fact, you may have taken a long break from dating because of them. (+0)

    b) The perfect door-holding, clean-mouthed, churchgoing person—or at least they seemed that way at first (+0)

    c) The reason you had to get treated for an STI (+0)

    d) Very vanilla—and you liked it that way. Leave the other thirty flavors for everyone else. (+0)

    e) Very adventurous (maybe more than you—which ain't easy!) (+1)

17. Would you let your partner stay in the room during your pelvic exam?

    a) Sure, why not? Nothing they haven't seen before (+2)

    b) Possibly (+1)

    c) No way (+0)

18. When you notice a slight increase in vaginal discharge, you:

    a) Add a harsh cleanser to your bathwater (+0)

    b) Douche (+1)

    c) Immediately call your gynecologist (+0)

    d) Monitor it for a few days before seeing a doctor (+4)

19. Which celebrity is most likely to pop up in your sexual fantasy?

    a) Adam Levine, Benicio del Toro, Nicki Minaj, Miley Cyrus (+2)

    b) Dwayne Johnson, Blake Shelton, Beyoncé, Gwyneth Paltrow (+1)

    c) Will Smith, Hugh Jackman, Jennifer Aniston (+1)

     d) Denzel Washington, Chris Pratt, Tom Cruise, Meghan Markle (+1)

     e) Ed Sheeran, Ryan Gosling, Eva Longoria, Gina Rodriguez (+0)

20. When you mention your vagina to someone, you're most likely to call it:

     a) Mention it? I don't. But I guess I'd say "down there" or "it." (+0)

     b) "Lady parts" or "vajayjay" (+1)

     c) "My vagina." It is what it is. (+2)

     d) My pussy, the Republic of Labia, cock sock, fun hatch—whatever! (+3)

Add 'Em Up

What's My V Personality?

If you scored between 0 and 10: Virgin Mary

If you scored between 11 and 18: Sanctified Snatch

If you scored between 19 and 27: Coochie-Chondriac

If you scored between 28 and 36: Mary Jane

If you scored more than 37: Notorious V.A.G.

INTRODUCING: YOUR VP

The Virgin Mary

Conservative, conscientious, quiet—that's you. What Nicki Minaj does in the daylight makes you blush, so imagining what goes on behind her closed doors in the dark would likely have you full-on fainting. Am I right?

While you don't have a lot of experience when it comes to sexual relationships, that means you don't waste a single second worrying about getting a sexually transmitted infection (STI) either. What you lack in bedroom bravado, you make up for with your nurturing temperament, laser-sharp focus in life, loyalty in relationships, and determination.

Friends and family might call you shy or an introvert. Your trepidation around sex could be due to your upbringing (it's how your momma taught you), or a bad sexual experience. There are often times when you consider breaking out of your shell, but you are also very comfortable in it. So even the strongest waves of FOMO (fear of missing out) can't catapult you out of your safe place. But you can't help but wonder, often, if you're truly living your best (sex) life.

The chances that you've grabbed a mirror to take a look down there are pretty slim to none. So this book is about to open up a whole new world to you. Buckle up, it's going to be an interesting (and absolutely essential) ride.

The Sanctified Snatch

You'll know you've landed in the right category if the name of this personality type ruffled each and every one of your feathers. But I need you to shake it off. As a former Sanctified Snatch, I know this VP intimately, so trust me: you're going to want to keep reading.

Kindhearted, reserved and, possibly, religious would describe you to a T. Chances are you've been called "prim and proper" before. It doesn't matter. You know exactly who you are: a woman with strong boundaries, strong beliefs, and strong faith. It's nobody's business whether or not you need to "clean up" after sex. You sometimes wonder, though, if you're keeping your partner in line or if you might be boring him.

You may not be as familiar with your body as other personality types. That makes communicating what you like to a partner (or explaining to a gyno what's wrong) very hard. But as you learn more about yourself in these pages, Ms. Goody-Goody, you might undergo a bit of a transformation.

The Coochie-Chondriac

I see you at my practice. All the time. (Girl, I said: *all the time.*) That's because Worry is your middle name. Whether you've been misinformed by someone, scarred by an experience with a partner, or getting a little too freaky too frequently with others, you're more anxious about the state of your V than the president is about the State of the Union.

Attentive to details, focused on health, and slightly self-conscious are the hallmarks of a Coochie-Chondriac. That combination can add up to some low-level anxiety, so anytime you notice a change in your discharge, your period's a day late, or you feel a quiver in your belly, you're booking an appointment with your gyno.

If your V could talk, its wish for you would be the same as mine: peace of mind. If you're constantly worried about what's happening to your vagina, you're stealing so much joy from your relationships. Instead of relaxing with a partner, you might be constantly suspicious of them. Instead of feeling free during sex, you might be feeling fearful.

I have a hunch you're ready to swap stress for serenity since you picked up this book in the first place. And I'm going to teach you how to do that by helping you recognize what's happening, build confidence in your body, and learn how to take control of your sexual health. (Oh, and you'll save a helluva lot on co-pays in the end too.)

The Mary Jane

I can spot a Mary Jane a mile away because, well, dame recognizes dame, and I'm definitely an MJ. We're dependable, classy, and idealistic. There are a lot of us out here. It's one of the most common VPs I see, so we truly are your average girl.

In relationships, MJs don't bring a lot of drama, but they also don't usually open the door to a lot of excitement. We're a cup of vanilla—not three scoops of rocky road in a cone. If a partner is looking for adventure, they should be aware that there's a roadblock here. If they're looking for stability, security, and safety—jackpot! They just hit the Mega Millions. That's what we're willing to provide because it's also what we crave.

The trouble is sometimes that stability leads to a partner losing inter- est. Actually, can we be real? Sometimes that stability leads to *you* losing interest.

Your friends probably call you a "great girl or a "good catch," and you definitely feel that way. You've got good intuition, you're honest and perceptive, but you're also wondering if there's more to explore when it comes to your sexuality. Chances are there is. As a fellow MJ, I'm going to fill you in on all that I wish I'd known about this personality type.

The Notorious V.A.G.

Mile-high club? Park after dark? Hotel rooftop? When it comes to sex, you've been there, done that, and you're not afraid to tell your girlfriends (or guy friends) all about it. You're adventurous, you're spontaneous, and you're in it to have an orgasmic time.

You stand out a bit because you tend to be the life of the party. People like you—but they're also afraid to *be like you*. Perhaps sometimes you're a little too loud. Or maybe you say things that can be embarrassing for a friend every once in a while. Regardless, you're not about to feel ashamed.

Of course, there are haters. Some women may be afraid that an extrovert like you will steal their partner. You've probably been called a "ho" before—but you know it's by someone who doesn't have half as much fun in their whole body as you do in your pinky toe. They can keep their labels while you're out here living, laughing, and loving it up. But there are precautions an NV needs to take and a ton of education she needs about whatever her life choices are—and that's where this book comes in.

There's no particular "look" for a Notorious V.A.G. She could be tall, short, skinny, voluptuous. Appearance doesn't matter, her skyrocketing confidence does—and she has more than enough to share with the rest of us.

5 Qs ABOUT YOUR VP

Q. I read the descriptions and I think I'm a different personality than my score. What's going on?

    A. Let me ask you something first: Were you absolutely, positively honest with all your answers? I'm going to ask you to go back and take a look at them again just to double-check. (We checked and double-checked the VP test as well, so don't take it personally.) In my practice, I've met Notorious V.A.G.s masquerading as Mary Janes and Virgin Marys pretending to be Sanctified Snatches. Sometimes the truth is tough to see. But if you really do think you fall into another category, in my professional opinion, you should go with your gut instead of your number. You know you best!

Q. Is it possible that I'm a combination of more than one personality?

A. Yes, ma'am. I'm a Mary Jane with a dash of Coochie-Chondriac. And I've definitely met Sanctified Snatches with a Notorious V.A.G. streak. I don't think that anyone is 100 percent anything. But there are also a few reasons why you might be a combination, like a recent change in your relationship status or a recent diagnosis from your doctor. If you feel like you overlap between categories—especially if your score was just a few points shy of another category—try to figure out which personality might be dominant over the other. Use that to guide your way through the book, but be sure to read through advice I have for both types.

Q. What exactly influences my VP?

A. Honestly, everything. I have to admit that nothing tickled me more than when I took this question to my Instagram followers and my phone started vibrating off the table with every response that came through. Here's what people were naming and claiming:

- "Zane books were my influence growing up."
- "Love and affection."
- "My upbringing."
- "An unforgettable trip to Paris that I took."
- "Television."
- "My boyfriend. There's nothing like being introduced to things you didn't do before."

I'm not going to lie to you, ladies: our sexual partners have an impact on our VPs. A big impact. How could they not? A partner can make you feel timid in bed or completely untamed. They can put you at risk or they can put you on a pedestal. But I was surprised that not a single solitary person responded to my post by saying "me." "Whatever I decide." Or "this chick right here." Remember that *you* choose your partner, so really the choice is in your hands. One more thing to hold fast to: the VP is only second-in-command. You're the commander in chief and you run your very own Oval Office.

Q. Great, but wait: How do I get a new VP if I don't like the one I have now?

A. The same way that you'd change any other aspect of your personality—like if you wanted to become less shy, a little bit funnier, a little less obsessive, or whatever. You've got to get out of your current comfort zone to move into another.

But to make it a bit easier, I came up with my top seven ways you can try to break into a new VP:

- **Schedule some sweat sessions.** No, not *those* kind. I'm talking about working out. You've seen me lifting weights, throwing punches, and doing box jumps on Instagram. Feeling more confident and in control of your body could be the boost you need. That physicality in the gym can impact your physicality in the bedroom. Whether you pick a routine like boxing (to feel powerful), Zumba (to feel sexy), yoga (to get flexible), or something in between, make sure it's something you find fun and can stick with.
- **Try meditation.** The body will go if the mind says so. If you can quiet those voices in your head that say "I have to be proper" or "what if my partner judges me" and hone in on the single voice that says "I want to free my V," well . . . you will.
- **Expand your crowd.** Instead of traveling in the same VP circles you usually do, try spending time with some other VPs in your

xxxii   INTRODUCTION

life at work, in your neighborhood, in your running group, or at your book club. Meet up with them for a happy hour or a night out at a club and watch what happens.

- **Open your eyes.** There's a reason why the *Fifty Shades of Grey* books made E. L. James an estimated $95 million. Use books and movies to take a look into the sex lives of others and pick and choose what you like.

- **Get out of town.** Travel somewhere by yourself and talk to strangers. It's easier to be the VP you want to be when nobody knows you!

- **Play the part.** Try a new sexual position, or open up to your OB-GYN more than you usually do. You might need to fake it until you make it. Think: What would a Notorious V.A.G. do? and just act like that VP until you get there!

- **Talk to a therapist.** You could be settled in your VP because of something difficult or possibly traumatic that happened in your past. It might take meeting with a therapist to work through that trauma so you can be the VP you want to be.

Q. How long does it take to change my VP?

   A. It can happen overnight (hopefully one hot, steamy, passionate night). You may wake up one day and find that it's changed based on your experience with a partner, a heart-to-heart with a friend, learning more about your body, or just a willingness to transform into another person. And don't be surprised if it changes as a result of reading this book right here.

HOW VPS REIGN IN THIS BOOK

VPs are basically the foundation for this book because, while I can *tell* you everything you need to know about your sexual health, each of you will *hear* that information differently—according to your VP's transla-tion. That's why, as you read each of the twelve principles I've laid out in this book, I'll have special messages sprinkled throughout for each VP. At the end of every chapter ("Point of V"), I'll also include overall takeaways that everyone should keep in mind.

What you're really going to love are all the absolutely true—and completely anonymous—stories that I'll be sharing about patients I've seen over the years. All names have been omitted to protect the inno-cent. Instead we're calling everyone by their VP name. That will help you imagine yourself in different sexual or healthcare scenarios you haven't encountered yet—or better navigate those situations the next time you do.

Point of V: Choose Your Own VP

Years ago, a Sanctified Snatch friend of mine almost turned into a Noto-rious V.A.G. After she had been spending time at home raising the kids while her husband brought home the bacon, they suddenly had a role reversal. He lost his job and she went back into the workforce to keep the family afloat. Not only was she a boss at work now, but she was also show-ing up to an office where an attractive colleague would compliment her. Every day she'd hear "that dress looks beautiful on you" or "your smile looks so lovely today" from the same colleague—who was inching her closer to the bedroom.

I've always said that you have to plant the seeds of what you want your harvest to be. This man was planting seeds for a relationship (clever guy). But, more important, my friend had expanded her crowd—one of the steps that can change your VP—by getting out of her home and working in an office. With every compliment, every smile, and every glance, this new guy was making her feel like the super-sexy girl she could be. She never had a physical affair with this man—she wasn't willing to sacrifice her happy family—but the emotional infidelity was the stuff they make movies about.

I'm telling you this story because I want you to know that you don't have to have an extramarital relationship to transform your VP. Had this Sanctified Snatch's husband been showering her with compliments—or had she been working on feeling sexy herself—the results could've been the same (well, with a lot less drama). Plant the seeds for the VP you want to be and get growing, girl.

THE
QUEEN

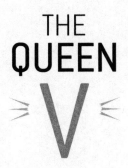

Don't Call It Wrong If You Don't Know What's Right

"THE MOST BEAUTIFUL VAGINA IN THE WORLD"

Every doctor has dealt with a funny little thing we call the "doorknob question." It's a question that comes up as soon as I'm about the leave the exam room. A patient will ask me one more thing they've been holding in—usually a bombshell—because they realize it's now or never. If they don't speak up in that moment, it'll be another six to twelve months until their next appointment.

As soon as I put my hand on the exam doorknob to leave, a Virgin Mary who's been working up the courage to ask about an unusual odor will say, "Dr. Jackie, can I ask you one more thing?" Or a Coochie-Chondriac who has already gone down a list of questions wants to ask me for the third time if I'm really sure that she doesn't need an STI test.

But over a decade ago, a Mary Jane patient of mine hit me with a "doorknob question" that was actually a "doorknob declaration." As I was about to leave the room so she could undress for her exam, this Southern transplant from up north wearing a St. John suit and perfectly matched shoes said, "I just want to let you know something, Dr. Jackie. I have the prettiest vagina you will ever meet. She's perfect in all ways."

I thought I'd heard everything—but never this. Especially not from a woman who had given birth twice and was in the first trimester of her third pregnancy. A woman who was actually here complaining about pain during sex.

I asked her what she meant by "perfect," and she broke down what made her lady parts the Marilyn Monroe of vaginas: the lips, the color, the symmetry, and, better yet, the smell. Who describes their vagina as smelling good? This woman right here. I've had patients say there was no smell. But to hear a woman say it smelled good was a first for me. I'm a straight, strictly-dickly woman. But let me tell you—at that moment I was very excited about seeing this patient's "perfect" vagina.

And here's what takes the cake: as a medical professional who has examined thousands of vaginas in her practice, I have to say that she was right. This was one close-to-perfect, cute coochie. To my amazement it had some of the best symmetry I'd ever seen, plump lips, and a perfectly acceptable aroma.

That appointment messed with my head so much I went home that night to see if my own coochie was as cute. But here's the catch: This Mary Jane wasn't looking for approval or confirmation during our exam. She was confident enough about her perfect-ten coochie that she didn't care whether or not I agreed. *And neither should you.*

While that's the kind of confidence you probably have to be born with, the rest of us can still (and should) strive to love what we've got between our legs for everything it does: giving pleasure, giving life, and more. And we certainly shouldn't judge our Queen Vs as being unattractive, smelly, or something to be ashamed of. The bottom line is that every V is truly beautiful, has a natural odor, and is something to be proud of.

But you can't love it if you don't look at it, don't talk about it, and don't know how it works. So let's start with getting to know your anatomy.

OUT OF SIGHT, OUT OF MIND

When was the last time you took a really good look down there? Probably when there was a problem. You noticed some discharge and wanted to get a look at the color. You felt some friction and wanted to make sure that bump wasn't more than a bump.

When I polled my Instagram following, a whopping 83 percent of women said they'd taken a glance at their Queen V. But that doesn't mean it was recently. (Ask any man and he'll tell you he gets a bird's-eye view and a good feel every time he goes to the bathroom.) I'm not saying you should do it every day, but ladies, if you can count on one hand the number of times you've looked, it's time to grab a mirror again.

To all my Virgin Marys and Sanctified Snatches out there, you may not have ever taken a look. For the Coochie-Chondriacs and Mary Janes out there, maybe fear or guilt has held you back. I'm here to free all of you from all of that by not only giving you permission to take a look, but also telling you that it's doctor's orders. Still not convinced? These are my five Ps as to why you must get more familiar with your V:

1. **Problems.** If you don't know what "normal" looks like for your vagina, how will you be able to tell when something looks "abnormal" or different?
2. **Praise.** How about a little appreciation for your vagina? You too could have the most beautiful vagina in the world. But if you never give it a second to sit in a spotlight (or just the light of your phone), you'll never know how it can shine!
3. **Pleasure.** And how about being able to ID what you're touching so you can tell your partner what you like? Sometimes when sex feels good, you don't know where that sensation is coming from. Taking a good look (or stroke or poke) down there will help.
4. **Prevention.** If you find something is amiss in your vulvovaginal area sooner rather than later, it could be the difference between life and death.
5. **Pride.** Knowing your body—what you love about it, what makes it feel good, what makes it beautiful—can bring confidence, acceptance, and, most of all, self-love.

So let's begin, shall we?

SEXUAL ANATOMY 101:
YOUR VULVA—LET'S CALL
HER YOUR VAGINAL FLOWER!

All right, ladies. Time to get naked. I want you to strip from the waist down and stand in front of a full-length mirror so you can get a frontal view of your mons pubis (it's the fleshy part of your body that cushions your pubic bone and is usually covered in pubic hair) and your vulva (the external organ that people usually think of when they say "vagina." Sometimes you may hear them called "lips"). In reality, your vagina is an internal organ, the canal between your vulva and your cervix (but we'll get to that later). Your vulva is made up of your:

- **Labia majora and labia minora.** If your labia were curtains covering the window of your vagina, these would be the outer and inner veils, respectively. The outer lips of your vagina (majora) are usually thick folds while the inner lips (minora) are thinner in texture. Together they're the gatekeepers to your vagina. Both protect the vagina from outside intruders like infections, irritation, and injury.
- **Urethral opening.** This is the gate to your bladder. It serves to keep urine in until you are ready to release it.
- **Vaginal opening.** It's the beginning of the vagina and near where the hymen lies. We lose this when we lose our virginity, have a rough fall on a bicycle, or experience some other type of trauma.
- **Clitoris.** Welcome to the command center of pleasure. It's the erectile tissue found anterior to the labia majora and above the urethral opening. It contains over eight thousand nerve endings.

The only constant in life is change. And that goes for your female sexy parts as well. All these sections of your vulva can shift due to different factors like:

- **Stimulation.** Much like with a man's penis, when you're sexually aroused, blood rushes to your clitoris and your labia, causing them to become enlarged. Once you reach climax, your organs will return to regular size.
- **Trauma.** Sex without enough lubrication, for example, can lead to a temporarily enlarged labia because they are swollen.
- **Weight gain.** Women who are morbidly obese, for instance, have a larger mons pubis as well as larger labia. This also occurs with weight gain due to pregnancy.
- **Illness.** A yeast infection or an allergic reaction, among other things, can lead to swollen labia.
- **Childbirth.** Vaginal delivery can cause the labia minora to stretch and tear, but most women heal within a few weeks.
- **Age.** Just like your triceps, the lips of your vagina can lose tone over time.
- **Hormones.** Taking large doses of testosterone can irreversibly enlarge your clitoris.

While no two vulvas are identical, I've noticed a lot of similarities among them from the other side of the stirrups. I ended up dividing the types of vulva into six different categories, which are all represented by a different type of flower: a rose, a sunflower, a tulip, an iris, a carnation, and a peace lily. Each shape differs according to what you can see of your vulva. Take a look in the mirror and then check this chart to see which vaginal flower reflects your vulva.

WHICH IS YOUR VAGINAL FLOWER?

1. The Rosebud

If you're flaunting this flower, it means that your labia majora and minora are doing exactly what they were designed to do: protecting the Queen V (your vagina). By the majora being closed and the minora neatly tucked inside you, your labia make it harder for anything unwanted to come in (or other things to go out) of your vaginal canal. If pornography was your primer on what vaginas look like, you probably think this buttoned-up beauty is pretty common and ideal. Actually, experts say it's fairly rare. This rose by any other name has been nicknamed "Barbie Doll" and "Fortune Cookie"—no surprise there.

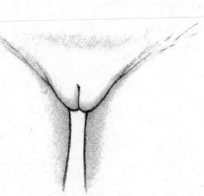

2. The Sunflower Petals

The defining feature for this vulva: labia majora shaped like a horseshoe pointing downward. That leaves the labia minora slightly exposed at the top, but not the bottom where the majora (or, as I call them here, each sunflower petal) come together again to touch. Despite the fact that it's more front and center to report for sexual duty, I haven't heard any patients say that having their clitoris more accessible increases pleasure during sex. It is just another lovely variation on a beautiful theme.

3. The Opening Tulip

If you've ever pulled on a tight pair of leggings or slipped into a bathing suit and noticed that you had a camel toe, this flower's for you. Because your majora's two lips (see what I did there?) are puffy, long, or dangling, they create a great divide for fabric to slip into. (If they're very prominent, they can make your gyno exam a little more complicated if you don't have an experienced doctor.) Your minora may be slightly exposed or they could be hidden. Speaking of great divides, there's another one in terms of how women react to this shape. Some find it frustrating and seek out cosmetic changes while others consider camel toe to be extremely sensual. There is even a company that makes "Party Pants" underwear that fake the look for those who aren't blessed with an Opening Tulip.

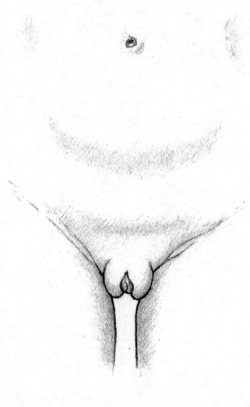

4. The Budding Iris

If you've ever seen a Georgia O'Keeffe painting, you probably expected to see this vaginal flower in the book. When the inner lips are starting to expose themselves outside the outer lips of the vagina, that's what I call a Budding Iris. This could be because your majora are spread more off to the side or are slightly shorter than the minora. Whatever the case, it leaves your clitoris prominently exposed, something I've heard patients complain about on occasion. But I reassure them that easy access to your ooh-ooh-ooh spot is a good thing.

5. Flourishing Carnation

Hello, spring! With this shape your labia are in full bloom, thanks to minora that are prominent, long, or dangling a bit. Remember, the labia are there for protection, so having them exposed means the mucous membranes can dry out. (Imagine how your eyes would feel if you never blinked!) Just try to take a little more time washing up (since they're so exposed) and during sex (so you're well lubricated and penetration isn't hindered). Wearing tight clothing might reveal an imprint of your carnation, but unless it's catching on your underwear (ouch!) or uncomfortable in regular activities, I tell women, "If your flower doesn't bother you, don't bother her."

6. Blossoming Peace Lily

None of us have bodies that are perfectly symmetrical. There are women who have one foot a half size larger than the other or one breast a cup size smaller than the other or, you guessed it, one labia larger than the other. Whether their minora are longer and dangle more on the right, their majora are less prominent on the left, or their labia are an unusual shape (like spiraled), asymmetry can make women feel unattractive and uncomfortable. The good news is that there is nothing wrong with these unique shapes, but if you choose to have them surgically modified, doctors offer plenty of options.

MIRROR, MIRROR ON THE . . . FLOOR

Now that you've gotten a good look up front, squat over a mirror or lie down on a bed with your knees back so you can see what I see when I begin an exam. In addition to all the parts of genitalia you saw before, you'll now be able to spot:

- The vaginal opening: the mouth of the vagina.
- The perineum: believe it or not, both men and women have a perineum. In women it is a nerve-enriched area between the anus and the opening of the vagina.
- The clitoris: this is the command center of pleasure. It looks like a penis but much smaller.
- The anus: an opening where your gastrointestinal (GI) tract ends. This is the last portion of the colon. Most call it an "exit only," but others may use it as an entrance to ecstasy.

Understand your norm based on its symmetry, color, appearance, any growths and, yes, odor. If there's a discharge or something coming from your vagina, as long as it's clear to white, it's normal, so there's no need to panic. Now that you know what's normal, let's talk a little bit about things you're concerned might be abnormal.

EX-QUEEF ME!

We've all been there. You're having hot and heavy penetrative sex with your partner when all of a sudden your vagina lets out a noise and you're mortified. (Did he or she hear that? Ugh!) It feels like the fart heard round the world. But, trust me, it's not and it's totally normal.

When your vagina makes a fart sound (or a vart or a queef as some people call them), it's not funky (like when you're passing gas), and it has nothing to do with what you ate (so keep the nachos coming). Your tooting is usually the result of pockets of air that were previously pushed up into your vagina getting released. No funk. No foul. Just the sound of freedom.

A Mary Jane I know has a husband who is not well endowed. She got a little frustrated during sex because his penis would frequently slip outside her while he was thrusting—and push air into her vagina as a result. She was basically living in Queef Central until she got creative with their sex positions. By straddling her man more often, she was able to control the action and reduce the slippage. Now all she does is rave about her multiple orgasms.

LUMPS AND BUMPS

I can already sense my Virgin Marys and my Sanctified Snatches tempted to skip over this section. Meanwhile my Coochie-Chondriacs are leaning in with two different colored highlighters. No matter which VP you are, I can't stress enough how important it is to protect your vagina by being able to put a name to anything strange and any abnormalities that can arise. These are seven of the most common causes for concern I hear from women:

Folliculitis

What it is: You'll feel this bump more than you'll see it. A quick inspection may show a small pink or large red lump or lumps on the labia majora or mons pubis. They're usually caused by bacteria in the hair follicle (from a pubic hair turning back into the hair shaft). It's time for a new razor, girl. These bumps are the bane of below-the-belt existence for African American women in particular because of our naturally curly hair.

Sometimes confused with: A painful herpetic lesion.

How to tell the difference: Folliculitis is more common around your period because of hormonal changes and usually resolves itself in a few days.

Protect yourself: Skip using dull razors or going to unlicensed wax salons. There is an art to hair removal and the extra dollars are worth avoiding this drama.

Treat yourself: These bumps will go away on their own, but if they don't in seven to ten days, see your doctor.

Fordyce Spots

What they are: A completely benign, incredibly common and non-contagious grouping of tiny spots that can appear on your labia when pores get clogged. They might be white, yellow, or red and are sometimes more easily seen if you stretch your skin apart a bit.

Sometimes confused with: Genital warts or skin cancer.

How to tell the difference: Let your doctor play detective on this one.

Protect yourself: This skin lesion is more common in oily skin types, so be aware of your norm and talk to your doctor about treatment.

Treat yourself: These spots often go away on their own, but it can sometimes take several years. If you want to speed up the process, talk to your doctor about surgical and laser treatments.

Cysts

What they are: Small, usually fluid-filled growths that can be a result of a blocked gland in the vagina (such as a Bartholin's gland cyst or sebaceous cyst) or trauma to the vaginal wall (such as an inclusion cyst, which may arise after childbirth).

Sometimes confused with: Skin cancer or herpes.

How to tell the difference: Many women talk about getting a painful cyst on their labia around their period. But once your period is gone, the cyst should be too. Better safe than sorry—have your MD check this out.

Protect yourself: Unfortunately, there's not much you can do to avoid getting a cyst in the first place.

Treat yourself: Leave these in your doctor's hands. They may decide to drain, remove, or biopsy the cyst once they've had a chance to examine you.

Skin Tags

What they are: Annoying but not harmful. These small, soft growths are often described as looking like a deflated balloon.

Sometimes confused with: Moles or genital warts. I have patients come in all the time who think (or hope) they have a skin tag, but I take one look at it with my naked eye or through a colposcope and confirm that it's actually HPV.

How to tell the difference: Here's another one for your MD. Book an appointment ASAP in case it is an STI.

Protect yourself: Experts aren't exactly sure what makes your body produce these pesky extensions, but they're researching everything from friction (places where your skin rubs together or against clothing) to genetics (you may just inherit them from Mom and Dad).

Treat yourself: While these growths sometimes fall off on their own, you can also talk to your doctor about having them removed by cryotherapy, cauterization, or surgery.

Genital Warts (See Principle #5)

What they are: Ridiculously common—so to all my Sanctified Snatches out there: please don't panic. Experts estimate that nearly every sexually active person will be infected in their lifetime with some type of HPV—the sexually transmitted infection that can cause genital warts and cervical cancer. They're raised, cauliflower-shaped growths that could be so small you can't see them or so large and clustered they're unsightly.

Sometimes confused with: Skin tags and Fordyce spots.

How to tell the difference: Aside from the unique shape of these growths, also consider if you've had a new sexual partner recently.

Protect yourself: As with all sexually transmitted infections, condom use can bring down rates of transmission. But you can expose yourself from skin-to-skin contact with a wart (outside a condom) as well.

Treat yourself: You'll need to see your doctor for management, which can be topical or surgical.

Genital Herpes (See Principle #5)

What it is: Blisters or sores caused by the herpes simplex virus (HSV), a sexually transmitted infection. They can itch, be painful, ooze, or even bleed.

Sometimes confused with: The results of a terrible grooming experience like a bad Brazilian, a painful ingrown hair bump, or a burn after leaving a chemical hair removal lotion on for too long.

How to tell the difference: Let your MD make the diagnosis, which they may need to take a swab to do.

Protect yourself: Always use condoms and avoid sexual contact if your partner shows symptoms of oral or genital herpes. You may want to channel your inner Notorious V.A.G., taking a bold look at a new partner in the light before you get busy in the dark.

Treat yourself: Your doctor can prescribe antiviral medications to help you heal faster or as a daily medication to help suppress the disease so you decrease your likelihood of passing it on to others.

Melanomas

What they are: Discolored lumps, sores, or thickening skin that are cancerous.

Sometimes confused with: Genital warts or moles.

How to tell the difference: Itching that won't stop; changes in size, shape, or color of a mole you've had for a while; an asymmetrical or large mole (bigger than a quarter inch). Experts have an easy way to remember what to look for by reminding you to think of the ABCDEs of melanoma: asymmetry, border irregularities, color that is not consistent, a diameter larger than 6 mm, and an evolution in appearance over time.

Protect yourself: Do regular visual inspections with a mirror and talk to your doctor as soon as you notice something wrong.

Treat yourself: We're talking about cancer, ladies. Do not delay talking to your doctor and getting treatment—it could save your life.

5 ANSWERS FOR YOUR DOCTOR

Every time I see a patient, I ask the date of her last period. And almost every time, the patient has to look it up on their phone, pull out a calendar, or just can't remember. Ladies, I need to ask you to be a little prepared for your OB-GYN visit. If you give me the information I need quickly, then we can get to the important stuff in your appointment a lot faster. When it comes to your last menstrual period (LMP), I need to know the first day it started with full flow, how many days it lasted, and how heavy it was (you can describe it in terms of tampons or pads used).

If you've spotted something amiss between your legs, be sure to have the answers to these questions so you can help your doctor help you. Think of them as the five Ws of lumps and bumps.

1. Where Exactly Is the Growth?

Be able to point to it and give your doctor directions (like "five o'clock" or "the bottom right").

2. When Did You First Notice It?

It might help to try to remember if it was there for your last period or the one before it. Or if there was a spin class you went to or a bikini you were getting into when it showed itself. You should also mention if it's uncomfortable or painful—that might've been your first sign that something was wrong. This information gives your doctor some clues as to what exactly the growth is and how aggressively it should be treated.

3. How Is It Changing?

Take a picture (just don't upload it to the "cloud"). Include an object (like a pencil eraser) for perspective and to check if it grows over time.

4. What Have You Done to Treat It at Home?

You know I want you coming to me first, but don't hesitate to fess up if you tried something over the counter or all natural that you found online. After all, if you've already tried something that didn't work, there's no need for us to give you a prescription for something similar. And if you tried something that added to the problem, I need to know.

5. Who or What Could Be Contributing to the Problem?

Has anything in your sexual health changed recently? Have you been with a new partner? Has your partner cheated on you? Have you changed detergents or body washes? Have you experienced any trauma like rough sex or falling off a bike? Any of these things could cause a reaction, expose you to a sexually transmitted infection, or result in an incorrect diagnosis (if your doctor doesn't know about them).

DESIGNER VAGINAS

"I hate my vagina," said a Mary Jane who came to see me over a decade ago for an annual exam. Part of my routine is to meet with patients with their clothes on so they can develop some level of comfort with me. Then I come back into the room for the physical exam. So when she told me she hated her large labia, I heard what she was saying. But I didn't fully understand until I got a look. Then I knew exactly what she meant.

This MJ's flower was an opening tulip with labia majora that were perfectly symmetrical but long and extremely large. Each one was the size of my hand, causing her to have to fold each labia into her underwear whenever she pulled up her panties. She had been to dozens of doctors who couldn't help her and, at the time, I was about to be another to add to the list. Back then no one was talking about "designer vaginas," much less essential reconstructive surgery on the vagina to ease the embarrassment, pain, and frustration of women like the Mary Jane I met. Now we do.

Nips, tucks, fillers, and tweaks down there are on the rise. From 2015 to 2016, there was a 39 percent increase in the number of surgeries done on labia by members of the American Board of Plastic Surgery. That's a lot of people tightening, toning, and touching up whatever makes them unhappy.

Numbers don't lie, but they also don't tell the full story. There's still a fair amount of research that needs to be done when it comes to how effective and successful vaginoplasty (a procedure designed to tighten the walls of the vaginal canal, often called "vaginal rejuvenation"), labiaplasty (cosmetic surgery to change the appearance of the labia minora), and labia majora surgery (just what it sounds like) are. But there's also a lot that we already know.

SHOULD YOU GO UNDER THE KNIFE?

If you're frustrated, uncomfortable, or in pain because of the way your vaginal flower is shaped, ladies, please pick up the phone and call your doctor.

A few concerns might rule you out for surgery right off the bat, like having a reproductive cancer or an autoimmune disease that could impact healing. It's also important to know that these procedures aren't covered by insurance unless medically necessary, so you may have to pay for them out of pocket. While you're waiting for that appointment with your doctor, ask yourself these four key questions to get the most out of your meeting:

1. Do I Want to Get Pregnant in the Future?

If so, surgery is not a great idea. Pregnancy and childbirth would only change your vagina again, causing you to need to repeat the surgery or making a vaginal birth more difficult.

2. How Is the Shape of My Vaginal Flower Hijacking My Physical Life?

"I wish my vagina were tighter," said one woman who wrote to me on Instagram. "But I'm appreciative that it hasn't had any issues or complications." She may not be a candidate for surgery. So who are the women who are? Ladies with skin tags painfully getting caught on the side of their underwear. Women who find swimsuit shopping an extra special nightmare because it's so hard to hide their labia inside their suit. Ladies who find having sex painful because of the way their labia twists, tugs, or get caught. Being able to express to your doctor what you'd like to change will help him or her figure out the best procedure for you.

3. Is My Flower Wrecking My Emotional Life?

One patient who came in to see me had labia minora in the shape of curlicue fries. Like an old-school telephone cord, you could pull it straight but it would curl right back up again. Take a second and just imagine what she must've been going through. On top of the physical problems caring for her flower, she was terribly embarrassed anytime she had sex. Your flower shouldn't interfere with your ability to have normal intimate relationships. It should enhance them. And just because you're at an appointment for a physical change doesn't mean you can't tell your doctor how something is hitting you emotionally.

4. What Complications from Surgery Could I Live With?

"My vagina is ugly," another woman wrote to me on Instagram. "I would change the inner lips if I could because they are too long. Then it would be beautiful." Perhaps true, but at what cost? While the vagina is very forgiving, it wasn't exactly meant for plastic surgery, and complications like loss of sensation, dryness, or scarring can arise. Solving one issue could float another one to the surface, so be sure to review all possible outcomes with your MD.

THE SPECIALIST'S CORNER: VAGINAL SURGERY

Whether you're thinking about giving your Queen V a makeover or already have a receptionist at your surgeon's office on speed dial, this advice from my colleague will be invaluable. John R. Miklos, MD, is an award-winning surgeon, a board-certified urogynecologist, and an internationally recognized expert in laparoscopic, reconstructive, and cosmetic vaginal surgery. Working out of Atlanta, Beverly Hills, and Dubai, his practices have treated tens of thousands of women. Here's our leg-crossing "V" Q&A on which procedure might be right for you, how to find the best surgeon, and the mistakes bad surgeons typically make.

Dr. Jackie: Give me your top three. What are the most common procedures women are asking for in your practice?

> **Dr. Miklos:** Number one on the list is labiaplasty minora. That's contouring and reduction in length of the labia minora. It helps patients who often complain that the protruding labia is not to their aesthetic liking and causes irritation when they wear jeans, fitted clothing, or tight undergarments. Next would be

vaginoplasty, which is when a surgeon tightens the inside and the opening of the vagina to enhance friction during intercourse. Third would be labiaplasty majora, where we reduce excess skin of the labia majora. Women who want this surgery are frustrated that their majora hangs when they're naked or looks bulky when they tuck it into a swimsuit.

Dr. Jackie: Any other honorable mentions?

Dr. Miklos: Clitoral hood reduction, where we decrease either the length or width of the clitoral hood, is fairly popular. This surgery can create a more symmetrical-looking vulva. Removing excess skin can also enhance sensitivity during stimulation of the clitoris. We also have women asking for the O-shot, which is an injection of plasma into the clitoris and G-spot to enhance sexual sensitivity and orgasm.

Dr. Jackie: What should a woman do before making an appointment for one of these surgeries?

Dr. Miklos: First and foremost, only consider doing these procedures if you're a truly informed consumer who understands the benefits and the risks of your surgery. You should also spend as much time researching your doctor as you do researching your next vacation. Probably more. Just like every figure skater or basketball player has their own strengths and weaknesses, no two surgeons are created equal either. When you're choosing a surgeon, evaluate them on four basic criteria—experience, expertise, reputation, and proof of skill, like before and after photos.

Dr. Jackie: Love it. How do you find a top-notch doc when it comes to experience?

Dr. Miklos: Ask them how often they do the procedure you're interested in. If the surgeon states, "I do these all the time," then he or she should be able to define that with numbers. One per year? One per month? Four procedures a week? If your surgeon does these "all the time," he or she should be able to give you the opportunity to have a discussion with his or her most recent patients. If the "recent patient" had her surgery twelve months ago, you really need to question your surgeon's experience.

Dr. Jackie: What about expertise?

Dr. Miklos: Ask them about their success rates and their rates of complications. Now, no surgeon can guarantee that you will be definitively tighter after a vaginoplasty, for example. Nor can he or she guarantee that you won't be too tight after the procedure. The most successful vaginal rejuvenation surgeons in the world have success rates of approximately 85–90 percent. That means approximately 10–15 percent of the time the procedure will not be successful—and success is determined by the woman receiving the surgery.

Dr. Jackie: Give me the scary stuff. What mistakes have you seen poorly trained surgeons make?

Dr. Miklos: One of the most common scenarios I see are patients who feel they look worse than they did before their labiaplasty. Sometimes they've had a complete amputation of the labia, and at that point, there's little I can do to help them. Another frequent occurrence is seeing patients who had vaginal tightening but the surgeon only tightened the vaginal opening. These women never have adequate results. The inside of the vagina as well as the opening needs to be tightened. This is why it is so important to question your surgeon as to their technique. No patient wants to go to surgery twice if it can be prevented.

Dr. Jackie: Can you do more than one procedure at a time?

Dr. Miklos: Yes. If a woman is discussing a lack of friction with intercourse, she should be prepared that her surgery might require more than just vaginal tightening, as many patients have an advanced condition known as vaginal prolapse that also needs to be treated. Women should understand that fixing the prolapse alone will not tighten their vagina.

Dr. Jackie: We both know there are risks to any surgery, but what are the benefits?

Dr. Miklos: Women tell me that they love their new vagina, that surgery changed their life and their activity level, and their sex life is back to being fantastic. Some women say their only regret is waiting so long to seek help.

POINT OF V: KNOW THYSELF

Whether you're a bold Notorious V.A.G. or a reserved Virgin Mary, you have got to get comfortable with your vagina. It's not silly, dirty, slutty, or strange to take a peek down there. It's necessary for your health. I know that will be harder for some of my VPs than for others. But, as I've already said, it's critical to know what's normal when it comes to your flower so you can figure out if and when things aren't normal. That familiarity means that my Coochie-Chondriacs out there won't freak over every minor change in discharge and my Mary Janes will have all the information they need to make their classic logical decision. Your vaginal flower has the power to make a huge impact on your life (for better or worse), so why not commit to getting to know her as soon as possible? Say, even putting down this book for a second right now to take a long, hard, loving look?

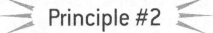

Principle #2

Vajacials Are Real—But You Only Need One Thing for Down There Care

UNFORTUNATELY, YOU'RE BEING VAGISHAMED

You may not realize it, but you're being vagishamed. That's what I call it when society tries to trick a woman into believing that her vagina is inherently unclean, unpleasant, unhealthy, or just plain bad. Ladies, it is not any of those things.

But just like talking about sex or simply whispering about masturbation, our culture perpetuates a negative stigma around the vagina. My Virgin Marys, Sanctified Snatches, and Coochie-Chondriacs probably already know what I mean. They find themselves paying extra attention to commercials that mention feminine odor. They spend hours lingering in drugstore aisles looking at products that promise to make them feel "fresher," "sexier," or (even worse) "more confident." They're constantly going to their gynecologist's office complaining of a musky odor—which is actually normal down there.

But they don't need to do any of that. And neither do you. Ask yourself: When was the last time you saw a man opening his wallet to buy something to help him feel fresher down there? Give me a break. Never. Not once. Unless they have a medical problem, men tend to leave their penises alone. (Let's be honest: when they do have a medical problem, unless it involves sex, they tend to leave it alone.) Meanwhile women are out here trying to set up at-home chemistry labs to test their vaginal pH.

The truth of the matter is that while you can do bad things *to* your vagina, it's *not* a bad place. And it certainly doesn't need an overflowing

bathroom shelf of products or a spa trip for a vajacial (see "What Exactly
Is a Vajacial" on page 32) to stay clean and fresh. Just like a self-cleaning
oven, your vagina has its own cleansing process thanks to the secretions
it releases. It also has a naturally balanced ecosystem made up of healthy
bacteria that you shouldn't disrupt. On a scale of 0 to 14, you want your
vagina's pH (the normal level of acidity present) to be between 3.8 and
4.5. Infections can change your vaginal pH, but so can your period, sex,
antibiotics, and hormones. Any chemicals you introduce into your vaginal
ecosystem could destroy its natural pH.

So if you want to save the Queen V, just use warm water to wash her.

Yes, you read that right: No gentle cleansers. No soaps. No specially
balanced body washes. No perfumes. None of that. I tell all my patients
not to let suds go past their clitoris and certainly not up inside the vagina.
Just use a soft cloth (or better yet, your hands) with warm water to cleanse
the folds of your vagina and the hood of your clitoris.

If you're worried the funk will fly every time you uncross your legs,
know this: there are a total of ten hygiene commandments I ask my
patients to follow. In addition to ditching soap, you need to stick to the
full list to keep your vaginal flower fresh as a sunflower, tulip, iris, carnation, peace lily, or rose.

THE 10 VAGINAL HYGIENE COMMANDMENTS

1. Thou Shalt Not Wear Silky Smooth Undies

More important than whether you're wearing a thong, bikini briefs, or
full-on granny panties is what they're made of. Cotton should be your
go-to material because it's breathable and will lower your chances of
getting an infection. Nylon and satin crotches feel luxurious but they're
breeding grounds for trouble because they hold moisture and bacteria
(save them for a special occasion when you know you won't have them
on for long). Finally, ditch your undies when you dive into bed. My
Notorious V.A.G.s out there are probably comfortable going commando

during the day (to avoid panty lines) *and* at night (to give your lady parts some time to breathe). As a Mary Jane, I'm not. Maybe I have a Juicy Lucy, but I don't trust my Queen V not to act out and leave a wet mark in the a.m. However, the nighttime is the right time for me to set her free.

2. Thou Shalt Practice the Pat-Down

You probably already know there's only one direction to wipe in after you urinate: front to back. Doing the reverse (back to front) risks pulling fecal matter and bacteria from your rectum into the vagina. As a result, you can end up coming to me with an infection. For some women though, it feels more natural to make that forward-sweeping motion. Others just forget when they're in a rush. One solution that can help: give yourself a pat-down instead of a clean sweep. After urinating, just take the toilet paper and push it into your urethra and vagina as if you're gently touching your face with blotting paper. You'll never wipe the wrong way again.

3. Remember to Pee Post-Sex

When your ooh-ooh-ooh-gasm is over, get up and go to the bathroom. It's a good idea for everyone and a mandate for any woman who is prone to urinary tract infections. The reason: when you're bumping uglies, unwanted bacteria can get up into your urethra and your vagina. But by going to the bathroom, you're helping to flush it out. In fact, one study found that a particular type of vaginal bacteria may be the cause of recurrent infections. Urinating after sex may help eliminate it.

4. Thou Shalt Not Soak More Than Shower

We all need to slip into the bathtub for a muscle-melting, luxurious soak every once in a while. But make sure you spend more time standing in the tub than you do sitting down in it. Marinating your V in perfumed, soapy, and dirty water ups your risk of vaginitis (see Commandments #6 and 10). Keep your soaks to once a week—if at all.

5. Thou Shalt Not Double Dip

Dear Notorious V.A.G.s: if you're trying to make sex twice as nice by having vaginal and anal intercourse in the same night, make sure you dip, pause, and then dip again. You need a quick intermission to get a new condom or have your man wash up in between. What happens in Vegas (your anus) needs to stay in Vegas. Don't let bacteria hitch a ride from Sin City to Reno (your vagina) just because you didn't want to ruin the moment. (The same holds true for the return trip.)

6. Honor Thy Aroma

Your vaginal flower might look like a tulip, but it's not designed to smell like one. So please stop trying to be a budding florist. Again, you're throwing off your vagina's pH. Skip the scented pads and tampons, deodorant sprays, and perfumes. Already have some on your shelf? Toss them right in the trash. Seriously. Right now. I'll wait.

7. Thou Shalt Not Douche. Period.

Every once in a while, a Sanctified Snatch or Virgin Mary patient will begin to tell me a story by saying, "When I douche—" I'll stop them by raising an eyebrow and a finger to say, "When you what?" It's the last thing I want you ladies to do, but it turns out up to 40 percent of women are still using these over-the-counter products to flush their vaginal canal with a cleansing solution. There are no proven health benefits to douching. None. There are, however, plenty of drawbacks: douches can push bacteria all the way to your cervix allowing it to travel to your fallopian tubes and your abdomen. This increases your risk of pelvic inflammatory disease (PID), pregnancy (if you've had unprotected sex), and more (see The Truth About Douches on page 30).

8. Thou Shalt Watch What You Eat

No one has funded a million-dollar research study on this, but it's generally accepted that bad foods for your lady parts are heavy spices, onions,
seafood, and—you saw this one coming—asparagus. I'm not telling you
to stop putting garlic on your pizza, avoid veggies, or skip eating fish, but
I am saying you may smell those things a second time if you do. That's an
odor—not an infection. It's something to be aware of if you're planning
on letting your partner go downtown, but it's not a reason to book an
appointment with me or any healthcare provider. The scent is completely
natural. Just let your partner know about the blooming onion you ate
before you slip into the sheets as a courtesy. You can also try to drink
extra water or eat sunflower seeds to flush out the scent. Never noticed an
odor? Turns out only 40 percent of people can smell the sulfur-like scent
their urine has after they eat asparagus. So even if you didn't sniff it, it
could still be happening.

Good foods for your flower include probiotic-rich Greek yogurt
(which can keep a healthy bacterial balance in your vagina) and soy
(which may help with vaginal dryness). Ever heard of Cum Punch? It's
basically fruits (like pineapple, papayas, and apples) men sometimes eat
to try to make their semen taste better. You can dive into a fruit salad
too to make a little Yum Punch for your partner. There's zero proof that
it works, but there's no harm in trying to make trip down south lead to
tropical waters.

9. Thou Shalt Not Be Alarmed by Totally Normal Discharge

I thought I'd crack up laughing every time a certain Coochie-Chondriac
patient came in and said, "Dr. Jackie, my monkey is funky—*again*." And
she came by a lot. She was absolutely convinced that her vaginal discharge
not only had an odor but that she and others could smell it when she
was in the bathroom, at church, and at her job. "I work with children,
Dr. Jackie," she said. "We have to fix this because if you smell, a kid will

tell you to your face." But they hadn't. Because she didn't. Clear or whitish fluid is completely normal. How much or how frequently it is expelled is different with each woman and can depend on where you are in your cycle or how old you are. As long as you don't have a truly pronounced odor, any irritation, or a thick or discolored discharge, there's nothing to worry about.

10. Thou Shalt Not Use Soap

Give your Queen V three weeks without soap and, trust me, you'll find her happier. If you can't imagine not using soap, just try it for one day to see how it feels. Then try a second day. Then see if you can make it to a week. Chances are you'll realize that you feel less dry, less itchy, and perhaps less irritated. If you absolutely have to put some sort of cleanser on, I'd recommend a small dab of 100 percent organic tea tree oil to kill odor. It has some sanitizing properties when placed on your skin—but it's not meant for areas with mucous membranes.

THE TRUTH ABOUT DOUCHES

Whether they're sitting on a toilet or crouching in the shower, every month millions of women are inserting a plastic nozzle inside their vaginal canal, squeezing it, and flushing their vaginas with a solution that promises to cleanse it. Sometimes it's a mixture of water and vinegar, sometimes it's other "natural" ingredients, but no matter what's in the bottle, I say the same thing: don't douche. The list of dangers tied to douching only continues to get longer. On top of risk of infection and pregnancy, new research shows that the process can increase your exposure to phthalates, a group of harmful chemicals—including one that has been linked to cancer and others that impact reproductive health. With all those drawbacks, I had to ask my Instagram followers why they continue to rinse and repeat down there.

Patients say: "That's what my mother taught me to do."

I say: "Momma didn't *always* know best."

And when she also told you not to mess around with that boy (you know the one I'm talking about), you didn't listen to her about that. So why this? My point is that times have changed and what we used to think was acceptable back then we'd never dream of doing right now. I'm here to officially make sure that you know better so you can do better by your V.

Patients say: "It makes me feel fresher."

I say: "It puts you at risk."

Just because nothing happened last time doesn't mean it won't happen next time. So many women chimed in to say they do it after their period or after sex—one of the worst times you could choose. You may have already introduced one foreign friend into your vagina that could carry with it a risk of infection, and now you're pushing that formula further inside you. Skip the floral flush.

Patients say: "My doctor told me to douche for bacterial vaginosis."

I say: "Are you sure? That's not what I tell my patients."

Because douching can alter the pH of your vagina and worsen the infection, I recommend prescription pills (like metronidazole or tinidazole), gels, or creams (like Clindamycin, Metrogel, or Nuvessa) instead.

Patients say: "It helps with the smell."

I say: "Cover-ups aren't a cure."

If you really have an infection that's causing a smell, you need a diagnosis from your gynecologist to figure out the cause. If your vaginal pH is off, they might suggest an over-the-counter gel like RepHresh to bring back balance. But if you're just uncomfortable with the normal scent of your vagina, spend a little more time researching eau de Vs to get more comfortable with it. The alternative could leave you with more problems than douching is worth.

WHAT EXACTLY IS A VAJACIAL?

The Coochie-Chondriacs reading this have probably already been there and spread for that—a few times. My Virgin Marys, on the other hand, are likely wondering what *in the world* is a vajacial! Short story: they're like facials for the part of your vulva (the outside of your vagina) that grows hair. Some salons only focus on exfoliating, moisturizing, and removing ingrown hairs from the area. Others add on high-frequency light treatment to eliminate bacteria or herb-infused steaming, where you crouch over a pot to "v-tox" your vagina.

Sounds invigorating, right? One Mary Jane told me: "It was a liberating experience because it stretched me out of my comfort zone." But a Notorious V.A.G. told me that it's not all that and a bag of herbs: "I basically sat on a toilet in a room with a bunch of other women to steam my vagina, hoping it would reward me later," she said. "It didn't." I'd warn you ladies not to book an appointment if you're looking for a miracle. While I've had patients claim that these treatments help with everything from infertility to menopause symptoms, pampering your privates doesn't go beyond a nice trip to the spa to deal with hairy situations.

I can't say that a little TLC for your vagina is a bad thing, but I also can't say it's a beneficial thing. There's simply no evidence to support that. If it makes you feel good (and look good), then I say go for it. Just make sure you use a reputable salon and let your OB-GYN know what you did at your next appointment. Always be as open and honest about everything you've done (from sexual partners to spa practices) so your MD can get the whole picture of what's going on in, around, and on top of your vagina.

GROW HAIR OR GO BARE?

I'll never forget the first time I saw a Notorious V.A.G. climb into the stirrups with her boyfriend's initials shaved into her pubic hair. I was speechless. She said it was a special treat for her man.

Since then, there's very little I haven't seen. I've had women open their gowns to reveal full-on Hollywood waxes with all hair removed, landing strips, postage stamps, arrows, and even a simple V. If you're up for carving crop circles into your own little field of dreams—or mowing the whole thing down—that's fine. But for one moment, I'd like you to step away from the wax or put down the shaving cream while I explain that your pubic hair has a purpose.

The same way that those tiny hairs in your nose filter the air that you breathe, your short-and-curlies shield you from bacteria and cushion you against friction that can cause skin abrasions. Somewhere over time, however, we got the idea that wall-to-wall carpeting doesn't look so good and we started opting for hardwood floors. Hair removal can get painful—and I'm not just talking about the sound you make after a strip of wax is pulled off. A shocking 3 percent of women end up in the ER as a result of genital trauma from grooming gone wrong. (Got 100 female Facebook friends? Three of them have a crazy ER story they're too afraid to tell you.)

I'm not saying that you have to leave your lady garden alone. A few Virgin Marys have shown up in my office with pubic hair so long I could've braided it! It actually inhibits my ability to do an exam if there's no clear pathway and I'm making my way through an untouched jungle, if you know what I mean. (It can also turn intercourse into, well, *inter-coarse*.) I just want to make sure you know there's no need to get overzealous mowing your lawn. Whether your down there hairstyle of choice is a Brazilian or a simple bikini trim, follow this grooming advice for happier trails. With all these techniques, placing a drop or two of 100 percent organic tea tree oil on the skin—not near mucous membranes—a day or so afterward can help soothe and decrease irritation in the area.

If You're Using Clippers . . .

Stop. While there are brands out there designed to remove genital hair, letting rotating blades anywhere near your bush (and your clitoris and your labia) is asking for trouble.

If You're Shaving . . .

Before you pick up your razor, shaving cream, or heart-shaped stencil, go get a mirror. Never shave blind. No matter how long you've known your Queen V, you still need a worm's-eye view from down below while grooming her to avoid an unfortunate accident. Soften the hair in the shower or with a warm, wet cloth for a few minutes. Softer hair is easier and faster to cut—think one pass, not two or three. Always use a fragrance-free shaving cream to avoid irritating chemicals and a new razor—so you don't have to worry about repeat runs down the same slope with an edge that's probably building up with dirt. Finally, shave downward, in the direction that your pubic hairs grow, to prevent ingrown hairs. Expect to be hair-free for about two or three days.

If you nick yourself, treat the cut immediately with Neosporin or another antibiotic cream. Letting bacteria into a wound can cause cellulitis, an infection leading to red, hot, swollen skin. Should this happen, or worse, head straight to your doctor.

If You're Using a Depilatory Cream . . .

As with any forest, the biggest concern here is fire. Burns can happen a few different ways with these creams and lotions that basically—poof!—dissolve your hair. If you go this removal route, make sure the product you've picked is safe for your genital area. Then ensure your skin won't have a reaction to the chemicals in the product by testing it on a less-sensitive area twenty-four hours beforehand. If you don't notice any darkening or irritation the next day, you're good to go. Finally, use the cream on clean, dry, hairy skin and watch the clock so you don't leave it on too long and get scorched. Expect your landscaping to last a little longer than shaving, from a couple of days to possibly a few weeks.

If You're Sugaring or Waxing . . .

You're a warrior queen. Period. These techniques pull hair out from the root—and sometimes tears out from your eyes. Sugaring sells itself as a slightly less painful and totally natural hair removal process that uses a single, sticky ball made up of water, sugar, and lemon juice to leave you fuzz-free. Technicians roll and remove the ball to pull out hairs. With waxing, technicians apply a thin layer of warm wax to the area, press paper strips on top of it, and quickly tear them off to pull out the hairs.

No matter which catch-and-release plan you choose, book your appointment at a licensed salon with licensed estheticians at least a week after your period. (You're less sensitive during that time.) Don't go in like a wooly bear either. Take some scissors and trim your hair down to a quarter of an inch or more. Finally, if you're getting waxed, don't let your technician double-dip by using the same tools (like a roller) on you that they do on other patients. You want to see disposable sticks and gloves or it's time to hop off that table. Because the wax can be hot, you could get a burn. Don't panic, just tell your technician. Use Neosporin or bacitracin on the area and see your doctor if you get a burn that is not healing properly. Expect results to last about a month.

If You're Going with Laser Hair Removal or Electrolysis . . .

You're looking for your Bermuda triangle to actually disappear, and with results that last anywhere for six months to forever, these pricey but effective techniques can deliver. Both treatments damage the hair follicles one by one using either a concentrated beam of light (laser) or shortwave radio frequency (electrolysis). While laser treatments delay or slow down hair growth, only electrolysis is considered to be the path to permanent hair removal. It's also better for all skin types (women of color generally need more treatments with laser hair removal) and hair colors (lasers look for pigment so they have trouble targeting gray hair).

5 VERY PRIVATE QUESTIONS YOU MIGHT BE TOO EMBARRASSED TO ASK

Q. I need the carpet to match the drapes. Is dying my pubic hair okay?

A. Getting rid of those fifty shades of gray isn't the only reason women want to color code their short-and-curlies. Some Notorious V.A.G.s want to go wild for Valentine's Day. Others just want the hair on their head to match the hair between their legs. Either way, harsh chemicals don't belong anywhere near your clitoris or beyond—neither does glitter—but if you insist on a technicolor bush, be careful. Don't let the product get anywhere near your mucous membranes, use a gentle formula specifically meant for pubic hair (like Betty Beauty or mini-KINI), and manicure your lawn after (not before) coloring. If you can, seek out a professional salon that specializes in this technique so you don't end up regretting your own attempt to throw shade.

Q. You said to cut back on baths, but what if I get the chance to jump in a Jacuzzi?

A. Live it up, girl! I mean, we're not talking every day, so have fun. Just be sure to put your hair up and take a quick shower with soap (but around your Queen V) before you put yourself on simmer. Everyone should. It helps eliminate the lotions, perfumes, and deodorants that can taint the water you're marinating in and also irritate your skin. (Yes, there are filters to clean the tub, but just like a major league baseball player, they're not going to catch everything.) Because there's a nasty little problem called Hot Tub Rash—a skin infection that can occur from being in a poorly maintained pool— you want to practice good hygiene once you're out of the tub too. Remove your bathing suit as soon as you can and wash up with soap (again, avoiding your Queen V) in the shower.

You'll avoid irritation that can come from any chemicals in the water lingering in your vaginal area and annoying yeast infections that can spring up from lounging too long in wet clothes.

Q. Back to that hot tub—do I have to worry about getting sexually transmitted infections in there?

A. No. What's more likely is contracting an STI from someone you decide to have sex with in the tub. What all those television sex scenes that rate 11 on a scale of 1 to 10 don't reveal is that chlorine and condoms don't mix. The chemicals decrease the effectiveness of your protection—and it's not like you're getting the tightest seal in the water anyway. Bottom line: Get playful poolside. Not in the water.

Q. I don't like how dark the skin is around my vagina. What do you think about labia bleaching?

A. I don't like it. Maybe the idea comes from watching pornography. Or maybe some of you have pushy boyfriends. I'm not sure where most women get the idea that they need to lighten their lips—or their anus—but every once in a while I have a patient ask me about it. In doctors' offices and the privacy of their own bathrooms, women are letting lasers and creams attempt to take their labia a few shades lighter. But that doesn't happen in my stirrups. Instead of equating darkness with being bad or unattractive, I want women to ask themselves, would they ever bleach a rose? Or slather lightening cream all over an iris? Let your vaginal flower bloom in its natural shade instead.

Q. Shapewear works wonders on my waist, but does it dethrone the Queen V?

A. It sure does—but I'm not going to tell you to never tuck in your spare tire. From first dates to weddings, at some point most of us need to squeeze into a twenty-first-century corset that leaves us waiting far too long to exhale. My one request: peel out of it as soon as you can. (I mean, we're all counting the minutes until we can do it anyway, right?) Compression garments create the perfect environment (hot, sweaty, tight) for breeding bacteria and are actually forceful enough to squeeze your internal organs. Bottom line: get in, get gorgeous, and get out.

THE SPECIALIST'S CORNER: PELVIC FLOOR HEALTH

We've covered your vaginal health in terms of how it looks and smells, but how about delving into how it feels? Turns out workouts aren't just for the muscles in your body that you can see. They're also for the ones you and your partner can feel. So I asked pelvic health expert Jennifer Hunt, PT, DPT, founder of Provenance Rehabilitation in Alpharetta, Georgia, for the 411 on Kegels, jade eggs, pelvic floor fitness, and more. Here's our "V" Q&A:

Dr. Jackie: Should all ladies be doing isolated pelvic floor exercises, like Kegels, every day to keep things "tight and right" down there?

Dr. Hunt: Not necessarily. Doing Kegels can make things worse for some women who have conditions like endometriosis or interstitial cystitis because they are often holding too much tension in their pelvic floor muscles already. In addition, many women can go their whole lives without doing a Kegel and never have a pelvic floor problem.

Dr. Jackie: What about sex? Can Kegels make your ooh-ooh-ooh feel even better?

Dr. Hunt: So there's no research supporting that. But my theory is that doing Kegels *correctly* helps women have better awareness of their pelvic muscles during sex—and that can lead to a better sexual experience.

Dr. Jackie: So all the hype we're seeing about jade eggs and other vaginal weights is just that? Hype?

> **Dr. Hunt:** Putting a weight in your vagina and seeing if you can walk around for an hour without it falling out is not a good activity for the pelvic floor. It can actually lead to pain or problems urinating by making it hard for you to relax those muscles. There are some pelvic floor gadgets that can be used appropriately though. If you don't mind spending the money and they motivate you to do necessary work, that's fine.

Dr. Jackie: Sounds like there are a lot of women doing Kegels incorrectly. How do you help them understand if they're doing them properly?

> **Dr. Hunt:** Imagine there is a marble at the vaginal (or anal) opening. While exhaling, you are going to try to grasp that marble and pull it up inside you using your pelvic floor muscles. Then, while inhaling, release the contraction as you imagine lowering the marble back to the vaginal opening and letting it go completely. If you insert a finger inside your vaginal canal and do a Kegel, you should feel pressure around your finger and an upward pull or lift of the pelvic floor. When women do the move incorrectly, they're usually squeezing their butt muscles or pushing down instead of pulling up. Also, it's a muscle contraction followed by a release of that contraction. Not a long-term hold. One more thing: it's not a good idea to perform these exercises while urinating or having a bowel movement. The pelvic floor muscles should be relaxed at these times.

Dr. Jackie: So who should be booking an appointment with you to come up with a schedule of exercises to do?

> **Dr. Hunt:** The most common reasons women come to me are painful intercourse, incontinence of any kind, pelvic pain, and

pelvic organ prolapse. In general, any woman who is experiencing any level of sexual dysfunction, bladder dysfunction, bowel dysfunction, or pelvic joint dysfunction should make an appointment. Educating women about what's normal and what's not normal is important.

Dr. Jackie: Let's tell women what some of the signs of dysfunction are.

Dr. Hunt: Sure. Any leaking of urine is not normal. Pain in the front of your pelvis while walking, climbing stairs, or just changing positions in bed is not normal. Frequent straining to have a bowel movement or feeling bloated is not normal. Going to the bathroom more than once in the middle of the night is not normal. Painful sex or not being able to have an orgasm is not normal.

Dr. Jackie: What kinds of exercises do you prescribe for women as a part of your personalized rehab programs?

Dr. Hunt: It depends on what they're doing the exercise for. Women experiencing incontinence, for example, might need to do squats and core strengthening. Women with pelvic pain may benefit from hip-opening stretches and breathing exercises.

Dr. Jackie: What should women know about booking an appointment with a pelvic floor physical therapist?

Dr. Hunt: They should have a clear understanding of what the examination is going to entail. I don't want there to be any surprise about what is involved in an internal pelvic floor muscle exam, meaning I will be inserting a finger inside the vagina to assess the tone and function of the pelvic floor muscles.

Dr. Jackie: What do you tell patients is bad for their pelvic floor health?

Dr. Hunt: One thing women might not recognize as detrimental is something I call JICing—that's going to the bathroom Just In Case. Voiding every time there's a toilet nearby can lead to frequent urination, urgency, or overactive bladder.

Dr. Jackie: How can you tell if you really have to go?

Dr. Hunt: I tell my clients about the 8 Mississippi Rule. If you can't count to 8 Mississippi while you're urinating, your bladder wasn't full enough for you to go. It's fine to have to urinate longer, but less than that might cause you to develop overactive bladder or urgency.

Dr. Jackie: Any other below-the-belt habits that aren't helpful?

Dr. Hunt: Staying in any one position for too long (standing or sitting). It's a detriment to the muscle balance of your pelvic floor—like always carrying your purse on your right shoulder. Chronic coughs, constipation, and holding your breath while lifting heavy weights can be harmful. Straining while urinating or having a bowel movement should be avoided. I know it's hard for busy women to do this, but take your time on the toilet, and if you frequently have difficult bowel movements, try propping your feet up on a Squatty Potty—a stool that puts you in the best position for going to the bathroom.

Dr. Jackie: And what are some good moves for pelvic floor health?

Dr. Hunt: Maintaining a healthy diet, drinking plenty of water, and being proactive—not reactive—when it comes to pelvic floor health. Don't wait until a problem gets bad. Respond immediately and try to prevent one from arising.

POINT OF V: GET BEYOND HAIRY SITUATIONS

It doesn't matter whether you're a Mary Jane or a Virgin Mary. Every woman reading this has very similar anatomical parts. Where we differ is in our levels of comfort in sharing and caring for them. My Notorious V.A.G.s will likely be more adventurous in their hygiene hijinks and go-to grooming of their Queen V. My Sanctified Snatches and Coochie-Chondriacs are likely more cautious and reserved when it comes to their techniques for keeping things clean, tight, and right. Regardless of your VP, my hope is that you've used this chapter to consider making over the way you keep your Queen V pristine. There's not a doubt in my mind that I surprised some of you with my no-soap solution to vaginal care. Yep, I stand by only using water. And you should too. But if that didn't make you say "Well, hold on a minute!" the fact that women are out here putting themselves at risk by douching or the realization that you're probably doing Kegels all wrong probably did. Take some time to revamp your old cleaning routine—and then stick to it to keep your Queen V safe, smelling normal, and ready for all the loving it deserves.

The Secret to Boosting Your Libido Isn't Usually in a Prescription Bottle

THE NEW SCIENCE OF LIBIDO

Sex drive. Desire. Sexual appetite. Lust. Sensual longing. The hots. Just like your Queen V, libido goes by many names—but experts are still working to understand that sensual force that makes us want to get it on. For decades researchers thought *spontaneous* sexual yearning was the norm. But some research now shows that one in three women rarely have an inkling to slip their hand over their husband's pants under a restaurant table or push up against their wife in a dark corner of the club. Here's the catch: even though they don't have that impetus, they often *do* respond (getting wet and excited) when those moves are made on them. So for every woman who has ever felt bad about herself because she didn't have impulsive sexual thoughts prompting her to action, research says you can stop feeling like there's something terribly strange about you right now. As part of 33 percent of the female population, you're definitely not in a small minority.

Experts also used to think that men *and* women followed the same sexual stimulus domino effect, going from desire ("I want to get me some of him/her!") to arousal (nipples hard, clitoris enlarged). But now we know that for many women, it takes arousal (getting those nipples hard, getting the clitoris enlarged) to *get* to desire ("I want to get me some of him/her"). That's why I often tell patients complaining of low desire to just go at it for a while with their partner and see how it feels. Some of us go from thirsty to quenched. Others get quenched and then it makes us thirsty.

Have I blown your mind yet? Well, keep reading because what I shared so far are two major ways our view of the spectrum of sexual desire has changed. Understanding the facts behind the fiction could change everything for you in the bedroom.

7 MYTHS ABOUT A WOMAN'S LIBIDO

1. Myth: Low Sex Drive Is Your Fault

Reality: It's a signal that something may be wrong, but this isn't a sign to start pointing fingers. I'll say that again because this is a really important point: **low sex drive isn't about placing blame.** Your Queen V is giving you a heads-up that there's a problem and you now have an opportunity to solve it. I do not want women thinking that it means they're broken, that they should feel guilty, that they need to come up with solutions on their own, or that they need to go to the doctor immediately.

Before we move on, I also want to say that women shouldn't think there's one definition of low sex drive. It's different for everyone. You can't just look at the national average of couples having sex one to two times a week to figure out if you're meeting a quota. If your sex drive is lower than what you've experienced in the past or if it's causing a problem for you or your partner, then you may have libido issues that are worth looking into.

2. Myth: Everyone Has Some Level of Sexual Desire

Reality: I've seen a few women who declare they just don't desire sex. A small, but still significant, 1 percent of the population defines themselves as asexual, meaning they lack sexual desire for or attraction to another person—even when stimulated. (For comparison's sake, 4.5 percent of Americans identify as lesbian, gay, bisexual, or transgender.) Before you jump to conclusions, let me explain that asexual men and women don't embrace this orientation because they had a traumatic sexual experience, they're not people who have decided to be celibate until marriage, and they're not individuals who just haven't found the right person yet. These men and women simply don't crave sexual stimulation.

That being said, an asexual person can still fall in love with someone of the opposite sex, want to spoon with someone of the same sex (but not "fork"), or both. There's just no desire to have intercourse. I have a married forty-year-old virgin patient right now, a bit of an SS, who has been with her husband for a decade and has never, ever, ever had sex. She and her husband sleep in the same bed, he doesn't complain, and they've never had kids. However, she assures me that they're happily married. (I'm frustrated just thinking about it, but they're completely fine!) Recognizing your own boundaries and being able to explain them to others can help you find the type of relationship you want to be in minus some drama.

3. Myth: Lack of Sexual Desire Isn't a Problem If You Don't Have a Partner

Reality: Oh really, single ladies? That's like telling yourself that not having an umbrella isn't a problem until it starts raining. It's true, but it's setting you up to end up all wet (in a bad way). You've also got to ask yourself the-chicken-and-the-egg questions: "Do I have low sexual desire because I don't have a partner? Or is the reason I don't have a partner because I have low sexual desire?" I see Sanctified Snatches and Virgin Marys who come from backgrounds where maintaining your virginity until marriage is extremely important. So they'll try to convince themselves they have low sexual desire as a way of maintaining their chastity. I had one of them tell me that she prayed God would take away her desire when she was single. Then when she got married and it still wasn't there, she said, "God, turn it back on! Turn it back on!"

4. Myth: We Should All Hail the Queen V as Our Most Important Sex Organ

Reality: There are many things we should praise your Queen V for, but being the most critical sex organ isn't one of them. Fun fact: it's your brain. (Yes, the mind truly is a terrible thing to waste.) There are women who can think themselves into an orgasm without so much as laying a finger anywhere on their bodies. What? Yes, baby, it's all in their minds.

Researchers have also been spending time looking at MRIs of women's brains while they're climaxing. The old thinking: a woman's brain shuts down when she has an orgasm. The new thinking: brain activity actually increases leading up to and peaks at orgasm, particularly tapping areas associated with pleasure (of course), reward, and addiction. Brain: 2. Vagina: 0.

One more thing: your skin is actually the largest organ of your body. Cue the baby oil, candle wax, or whatever you're into. It's the place for sensual stimulation from tickling and teasing to stroking and gentle spanking. Bottom line: despite the fact that your Queen V is often the bull's-eye your partner is aiming for, it's actually your brain that's the center circle.

5. Myth: Aphrodisiacs Don't Really Work

Reality: Sometimes they do. Feeling showered with affection because your man splurged on oysters at dinner and genuinely believing that slurping them up will spike your desire can have an impact. It's a little something called the placebo effect. When researchers were trying to figure out if the erectile dysfunction drug Viagra worked in women, some study participants got the little blue pill while others got a fake sugar pill. Turned out 40 percent of the women who got the sugar pill reported an increase in sexual desire. Similar results happened when researchers were looking at the placebo effect on another erectile dysfunction drug, Cialis, in women. Long story short: if you build it (up in your mind), you will come.

6. Myth: Libido Declines with Age

Reality: Some research shows it can actually increase. And let's also not forget all the other factors that contribute to your desire to get it on, like hormonal fluctuations (women who menstruate are randier midcycle when they're ovulating than right before their period), medications that can sap your desire (like certain antidepressants), lifestyle habits (drinking too much, smoking, doing drugs), feeling stressed (new boss at work got you down?), being exhausted (what does eight hours of sleep feel like again?), and more. For women, a lot more factors impact libido than just another birthday rolling in.

7. Myth: Having a Low Sex Drive Is Rare

Experts say as many as 80 percent of women will experience a low sex drive at some point in their lives—and for each of them the solutions to the problem will be different. But all too often, women think there's one solution and they can only get it by walking out of their doctor's office with a prescription. The answer is frustratingly more complicated yet far easier than you might think. It's also one of the biggest misconceptions about women and sex drive. So let's take some time to explore it.

FROM THE SAHARA DESERT
TO THE MISSISSIPPI RIVER

Years ago, a Coochie-Chondriac started coming into my office so often she practically paid for my Mercedes-Benz with her visits. She was thirty-eight, had been married eight years, had given birth to one kid, and— here's the frequent-flyer fiasco—had zero sex drive.

I ran all the standard tests to make sure that her estrogen, testosterone, and progesterone hadn't suddenly taken a dive. They hadn't. We went over her medical history and I asked her about any drugs she might be taking that could be the cause. There weren't any red flags. I sent her to a specialist to see if there was low blood flow to her clitoris or some other physical problem that was preventing her juices from flowing. There wasn't. I referred her and her husband to a sex therapist to see if that doctor had any ideas. She didn't. So month after month, with her husband's insisting, the Coochie-Chondriac kept coming back with the same complaint. "Something is wrong," she said. "Maybe you're missing what it is." But it wasn't me that was missing something. It was her.

There's a certain glow that comes over a woman who is happy in a relationship. This Coochie-Chondriac didn't have it. When I'd ask her about her partner, she'd just say, "He's all right." *Hmmmmm.* So, it was no shock to me when she came in one day and told me she was having an affair and now getting a divorce. (One of her husband's friends had caught her with her boo at a restaurant. She tried to hide underneath the table but it didn't work.) Here's the real shocker: she'd met a man at work who turned her on so much she'd feel wetness running down her thigh just being near him. While her dry marriage was over, she was on her way to getting hitched to the new guy who drove her wild.

VPS AND LOW SEX DRIVE

When patients come to me with what they call "decreased libido" or "low sex drive," nine times out of ten they're misdiagnosing themselves. (Just like those researchers I told you about, regular folks get things wrong too.) So often, women think they have a physical problem like a hormonal imbalance, but instead they're a Mary Jane who is so focused on being a working woman, "momager" (CEO of managing the kids), or "wifager" (CEO of managing her partner's life), that she barely has any energy leftover to be a "sexager." MJs devote so much energy to worrying about other people outside the bedroom that doing it inside the bedroom probably feels like *one more chore.*

Or they're a Sanctified Snatch who might see sex as more of a turn-off than a turn-on because she thinks it's unclean or just for procreation. But if she could put aside religious thinking for a second and loosen up, she just might get herself feeling, well, differently inclined.

And, of course, there are Coochie-Chondriacs, like the one who was up in my office on a monthly basis until she met the man who turned her Queen V from the Sahara Desert into the Mississippi River. For them, the real problem is that something is making them feel uninterested in, unattracted to, or used by their partner. Where is the love? Not in her relationship.

And in case you're wondering, my Notorious V.A.G.s and—surprise, surprise—my Virgin Marys are usually on point when they come to me with a libido problem. As a master of sexual expression, NVs tend to have an increased sex drive, so if something were wrong with her enthusiasm in the sack, she'd notice and act on it right away. As a master of sexual control, the Virgin Mary might have a high or normal sex drive, but she's taming the lion between her legs because she might be insecure, shy, or saving it for marriage. VMs may not be having regular sex with a partner—but that doesn't mean they're not having sex or noticing when something is off.

If you experience low libido, it's possible for your desire to amp back up when you solve a bigger issue that cropped up *outside* the bedroom. Some women have a sex drive that is in park *not* because their car has a legitimate mechanical problem (like a broken starter) but because of a user error (like someone forgetting to put high-octane gas in the tank).

I don't always have time to take off my lab coat and pick up my therapist pad and pencil during a patient appointment. So instead, I usually slip in a few questions during the examination that basically tell me which camp you're in. You can figure out the same by asking yourself these three questions—just swear to tell the truth, the whole truth, and nothing but the truth, so help your Queen V.

NO SEXUAL APPETITE? MAYBE YOU'RE HUNGRY FOR SOMETHING ELSE

Libido is obviously a little easier to judge when you're in a relationship, but my single ladies can ask themselves these three questions to see if their drive is down.

1. What Did You Think of That Steamy Sex Scene on *Power/Outlander/ Orange Is the New Black* Last Season?

If you don't find yourself whispering "I love you" to the television when Omari Hardwick graces your screen, maybe you do when David Beckham, Michelle Rodriguez, or Laverne Cox makes an appearance. Doesn't matter who the hot-hot-hot actor is that you've voted Most Likely to Get It From You in Five Seconds Flat. All I care about is whether your brain starts imagining exactly what you'd do to them (or better yet, let them do to you) if you got the chance. If so, libido isn't a problem. It sounds like your pipes are just fine but you need to show your partner how to turn your faucet on.

2. Can You Get Your Ooh-Ooh-Ooh on When You Masturbate?

You can do the math on this one. If you + sex = orgasm, that's great. But if you + your partner + sex ≠ orgasm, we know what's throwing an anticlimactic kink into that equation. If you've never engaged in a little ménage à moi, don't worry. I'm not judging you and you're not alone. While my Notorious V.A.G.s, Mary Janes, and Coochie-Chondriacs wouldn't hesitate to take matters into their own hands—whether they're in a relationship or not—my Virgin Marys and Sanctified Snatches were likely brought up to believe that masturbation isn't proper. Here's the problem with that: aside from the fact that you're putting all the responsibility of sexual pleasure on your partner, you're also shutting yourself off from sexual discovery that can help you teach your partner how to satisfy you. A little blue (or pink) pill won't show you what you like in bed. A little self-exploration will.

3. When You Have Sex, Is It Any Good?

I get a few different answers to this question. One response is a flat-out "Nope. I'd rather be sleeping." Then we know what the real problem is. I've also heard: "I don't know because it's not happening." There's only one way to find out. I tell my patients to try it. Some women need to have sex in order to feel like having sex. Not the other way around.

I've also had patients tell me, "It starts out good, but then goes downhill." It could be that you can't stop thinking about fixing your credit score so you two can get a new house. You're preoccupied by the idea of waking up early to avoid a scowl from your boss if you stroll in late. Your brain's sending the hot-and-bothered message throughout your body, but you're drowning it out with your #lifegoals. Your partner can help you relax and ramp up more (see the Four S's below), but you also need to put sex (not getting to Target first thing on Saturday to beat the crowds) at the top of your to-do list.

If you answered yes to two out of these three questions, then the problem is less low libido and more something I call a Vitamin S Deficiency.

HAVE YOU HAD YOUR VITAMIN S TODAY?

When I asked my Instagram followers what they want (but aren't getting) in their relationship, the responses came fast and (unfortunately, sometimes) furiously. You told me you weren't getting attention, communication, appreciation, time, affection, respect, assurance, compassion, and more. No matter what they DM'd me, the responses all fit into a few categories of things that every woman needs to feel loved and passionate in her relationship. I've heard Steve Harvey talk about these needs as the three P's. I like to think about them as the Four S's instead. When you get your full four doses of Vitamin S, you don't need to worry about the E and the X. That, ahem, comes easy.

The First "S" Is to "Say It"

Does your partner look deep into your eyes and say, "Baby, I love you"? Does he bring you out to meet his friends and make a point of introducing you as his girlfriend or wife? Does she roll over in bed, look at you when your hair is all a mess, and whisper, "You're absolutely gorgeous"? Maybe these affirmations have slipped through the cracks because you and your partner have been together for soooo long. Or maybe you never heard them in the first place. But having someone who consistently declares what you mean to them and announces it to the world is what so many women who walk through the door to my office really need. If your partner's not saying it, your Queen V isn't hearing it—so she can't respond.

If you're starting to get uncomfortable realizing that you're sleeping with someone who hasn't given you a title or simply paid you a nicety in darn near a month, don't get upset. Rejection is oftentimes for our protection. You can work through issues by asking for what you need. But if you have to force a relationship, it's not supposed to be.

The Second "S" Is "Safety"

We're not damsels in distress who need to be rescued. I think all of us have rewritten that fairy tale. Still, it's sexy when someone tries to take care of us. Maybe he shoots you a text at the end of the evening to make sure you got home all right. Or she makes sure that you have enough gas in your car and the tires aren't looking low. These aren't just reassurances of how much your partner is into you, they're also turn-ons.

Some shows of safety are about what your partner is willing to do for you. Others are about what they're willing to say about you. Ask yourself if your partner stands up for you when someone says something negative about you, whether it's their momma, their best friend, or a clerk at a store giving you an extra dose of attitude. A partner who truly cares for you will protect you from insults, injury, and inconveniences of all kinds. And your Queen V notices it all.

The Third "S" Is Financial "Security"

You know what can sap all the sexy out of a woman? Worrying all by herself about whether or not you can afford to go on vacation this summer, how you're going to make the next car payment, or what will happen if you get fired tomorrow. Even if you make more money than your partner and even if you're a better money manager than they are, you shouldn't be the only one stressing about the bills (and vice versa). You both need to understand the financial workings of your relationship.

If your partner doesn't know a 401(k) from a 529 plan, he or she can still express an interest in what's happening without having to do any heavy lifting. Just sitting down with you while you're working on the family bills or asking you how cash is flowing can make a difference. This can make you soooo moist.

The Fourth "S" Is a "Sacrificial Offering"

Early in my medical career when I had to work late nights and then walk to the hospital's parking garage by myself, Curtis insisted that I call him to check in. "Just wake me up and tell me you're leaving," he'd say. It would've been easier to sleep through the night, but he'd rather lose some rest to know that I was all right.

What is your partner willing to give up for you? Would he sacrifice trying to get ahead at work so you two can have a date night or a weekend away from his corporate email? Would she tell her best friends she can't hang out because she needs time to catch up with you at home? Does he say nothing but good things about you when you go to visit his family—even though you had a fight in the car on the way there? The partner who will put you first—even if it means a pain point for them—is the ultimate. Do you hear me? That's a true test for love.

TALLYING UP THE FOUR S'S

As you evaluate your partner, you also have to weigh how genuine their actions are. A Sanctified Snatch patient of mine had a husband who knew how to "Say It." He regularly told his friends and coworkers how much he catered to, looked out for, and loved her. But it was all for show. When they were behind closed doors, he basically ignored her. She didn't have a voice in their relationship and whatever he said went! Every time he professed his love for her in public, she wanted to call him a liar to his face right then and there—but didn't. (Consider this *her* sacrificial offering.)

One last note: the Four S's aren't a list that you put a check next to as your man does each one and call four for four a victory. Think of them more like quarters of a love pie. Your man might be giving you 10 percent security but 25 percent of everything else for a total of 85 percent of the S's. The goal is to get as close as possible to 100 percent. Anything less than 50 percent and you've got some work to do in your relationships.

INTENTIONAL LOVING: GETTING ALL THE S YOU WANT

So now you know what you need—and that you're not going to find it at your local pharmacy. The next question is how do you up your Vitamin S intake so you can get back to enjoying some ooh-ooh-ooh? You get your dose through something I call Intentional Loving.

Unfortunately, a lot of us know what *Un*intentional Loving looks like. It's the relationship where you let life happen to you rather than deciding what you two want out of life and going for it. It's the person who stands you up on dates over and over because "something came up." It's the person who is inconsistent in their actions—like not calling you every night before bed. As women, we often settle for Unintentional Loving and it's not until it's almost too late that we wake up and realize the tragedy of our circumstances.

You can be married and experience Unintentional Loving. I'm going to tell you something that not even my husband knows. Last year I bought Curtis a beautiful card and an expensive pair of sunglasses for Valentine's Day—but I never gave them to him. When I got home after a long day at work, Curtis and I had a nice dinner together . . . and that was it. I asked him where my card and my present were, but he didn't have a single thing for me but a surprised look on his face.

It would've been easy to keep the peace and just have a happy Valentine's Day. But I've been through too much counseling for that mess. We all know you have to teach people how to treat you, ladies. It wasn't fun and it didn't feel good, but I let Curtis know what my expectations were and that he'd let me down. Then I put his card and his gift—part of my gesture toward Intentional Loving—right back in my dang bag. He never saw them.

So what is Intentional Loving? It's something that gives your relationship a purpose and goals that you two are working toward. The Four S's are the foundation for the much bigger thing that you two are creating. Most people don't practice Intentional Loving because they haven't been taught it, they don't know how to make it happen or it feels too hard. The pain associated with not doing it is greater than the work that it takes to do it. But I think deciding to love intentionally is actually quite easy.

First, Decide What You Want

A partner who makes you feel safe? Someone who sets up date nights and vacations for you two to go on? A mate who showers you with affection? For me, one of the things I wanted was a partner who made sure to spend quality time with me.

Next, Define What That Looks Like

Him picking up the kids after school so you can hit the gym? Her texting you words of encouragement every day? Him sending you flowers every week? In my marriage, Curtis and I make sure that after church on Sundays, we do brunch together, and we really look forward to those times.

Then, Come Up with a Plan for Making It Happen

Maybe you've never asked for exactly what you want and it's time to tell the person what you need. Maybe there's a compromise that needs to take place. For Curtis and me, that means saying "no" to friends who invite us out on Sunday afternoons and trying to arrange my schedule so I'm often not on call that day.

Finally, Focus on Why It Will Be Worth Living This Way

Because you want to model what healthy love looks like for your kids? Because you're a power couple on the verge of creating an empire? For me it's about being happy, healthy, and wealthy. Pure and simple.

THE SPECIALIST'S CORNER: SEX THERAPY, PART 1

When a physical workup doesn't reveal the cause of a patient's libido frustrations, I refer them for counseling with a sex therapist. My go-to problem solver is Tiffanie Davis Henry, PhD, a certified sex therapist and relationship expert in Atlanta, Georgia. Here's our "V" Q&A on sexual blinders, your junior high relationships, and what everyone gets wrong about seeing a sex therapist:

Dr. Jackie: When men and women dial your number, what are some of the reasons they're booking an appointment with you?

> **Dr. Tiffanie:** Hands down, low sexual desire is the number one reason for women. About eighty percent of women at some point in their lives will experience low sex desire. What comes next would be relationship issues causing sexual dysfunction and then inability to orgasm. I've also had several "forty-year-old virgins." Perhaps they abstained for religious reasons, then no one wanted the responsibility of being their first in their twenties or thirties. Now they find themselves unmarried and just want to get it over with. And the opposite: women and men who have gone for a long time without sex because they're "born again virgins," had a sexual trauma, or haven't felt sexual in a long time.

Dr. Jackie: What have you noticed about sex problems in your years of practice?

> **Dr. Tiffanie:** Very often sex problems are a symptom rather than the actual disease. For example, difficulty orgasming is about letting go for many women. So when I'm working with people who say I've never had one or only had them via self-stimulation, I'll ask, "Do you have trouble letting go in other areas of your life? Do you feel like you have to be in charge all the time? Are

you able to delegate?" So we work on how to let go in other areas of their lives. Usually once they can master that, it's easier to let go in the bedroom.

Dr. Jackie: Do you also see a lot of women with emotional libido issues rather than physical ones?

> **Dr. Tiffanie:** Absolutely. Relationship challenges can cause a lot of emotional distress leading to issues with your libido. For example, I've seen married women who feel like single moms. They'll say, "My husband is very condescending" or "He doesn't respect my contribution to the household" or "We're arguing all the time." If you don't like the person you're having sex with, you don't want to have sex with them. Your brain is telling you something, but sometimes we expect our body to act in a way other than it should.

Dr. Jackie: Why do we put those sexual blinders on and only see what's right in front of us—this person we're *supposed* to have sex with?

> **Dr. Tiffanie:** It's the "should" statements we tell ourselves as women. I see women who are having sex as a means of checking it off a list of things they *should* do but not because it's something they really *want* to do. They think, "I should be having sex a certain number of times a week." Or their mother told them, "If you don't have sex with him, he'll get it somewhere else." We set standards for ourselves or our partners set them, then we question our ability to perform sexually when in actuality we're performing exactly how we are.

Dr. Jackie: What's standard operating procedure for the types of questions you ask patients?

> **Dr. Tiffanie:** I need to know what their level of sexual desire is. I'll always ask about verbal, mental, or sexual abuse they may

have experienced themselves, witnessed, or been exposed to in
some other way. I do an entire health history, physically and in
regard to relationships. Yes, I need to know who you dated in
junior high, for example. And then I ask what they'd like to see
changed by the end of this process and what has prevented that
change from happening up until now.

**Dr. Jackie: Okay, that's what *really* happens behind closed doors with
you. But what do most people *think* goes on? Any misconceptions about
seeing a sex therapist?**

> **Dr. Tiffanie:** I'm not watching you have sex. It's talk therapy with
> someone who is a trained mental health clinician with an exper-
> tise in sexuality issues. Also, some people think because I'm a sex
> therapist, my sex life must be kinky. I'm a normal human being
> like everyone else and what I do and don't do is my personal
> business.

**Dr. Jackie: What do people need to know before they go to a therapy
session with you?**

> **Dr. Tiffanie:** I get patients who say, "I don't want to have sex, but
> I want to want to have it." And then there are patients who
> say, "If I never have sex again, I'll be just fine"—even though
> they're there with a partner. Be honest about why you're there
> and what you want to get out of it. If you're coming with
> your partner, make sure you're on the same page. Also, know
> that sex therapy is a marathon and not a sprint. You've spent
> your entire life in this body and a lifetime coming into your
> sexual self. It'll take time to figure out what's causing the
> kinks.

WHEN THE PROBLEM IS MEDICAL

If you've gotten this far in the chapter and you're still saying, "Dr. Jackie, I know my problem is medical and not mental," then you're probably right. If we've ruled out a low libido tied to your partner, your relationship, or how you're feeling about yourself, it's time to analyze the potential chemistry behind your coital crash. Ask yourself if one of these issues might be the root of the problem.

Antihistamines

You wanted your nose to stop running—but you didn't want to have trouble getting wet down there. The problem is, your antihistamine doesn't know the difference when it's trying to dry you out. Luckily using a little lube until you feel better is a smooth solution.

Anxiety or Depression

Besides simply not being in the mood, medication you take to treat these mood disorders could impact how much you want to get it on. One side effect of certain antidepressants (like selective serotonin reuptake inhibitors, or SSRIs) has been found to be lower sex drive. The idea isn't to stop, but if there's cause for concern ask your doctor if you can switch to a different medication.

Birth Control Pills

Just like the plot of your favorite nighttime drama, one day research says birth control pills are good, the next day they're bad, the next day they're back to wearing a halo, the next day they've got horns. A pretty exhaustive study, however, found that it's a little more complicated than that. Even though these little pills can level out your hormones—so you don't get that randy spike in testosterone around ovulation—it turns out most women don't experience any change or actually have an increase in sex drive while using oral contraceptives. About 15 percent of women, however, do see their desire take a downturn when they go on birth control. Thankfully, there are so many different types of oral contraceptives on the market to switch to if you and your doctor want to try to counteract that impact.

Cardiovascular Disease

After surviving a heart attack, heart failure, or another form of the disease, it could be tough for anyone to feel carefree getting a workout in bed. You might be worried about triggering an event. Hypertension is considered a silent illness, so you may not realize you have high blood pressure or that it could be impacting your sex life. Full disclosure: the jury is in full agreement on how hypertension impacts men, but it's still out on how it impacts women. The theory is that it may lead to decreased blood flow to the vagina, dryness, and difficulty achieving orgasm.

Diabetes

Nearly fifteen million women in the United States have diabetes—and nearly 25 percent of them don't know it. The illness can impact your love life by decreasing blood flow to your vaginal flower or causing nerve damage. You might have low sexual desire, no sexual response, or decreased amount of lubrication in your vagina, as a result.

Pregnancy, Postpartum, and Menopause (Vaginal Dryness)

You're feeling nauseous, you're exhausted, your boobs are sensitive, and you're not loving looking in the mirror—but you're still wondering where your libido went? Then blame your shifting hormones—even after you deliver. The hormone prolactin does double duty on you, helping to produce breast milk but also leading to a dip in sex drive.

It's a similar story with perimenopause and menopause, when you're going through hot flashes, mood swings, and night sweats. Not exactly a "come ravish me now" combination. Point to those pesky hormones again, as your decrease in estrogen is sparking all this change, with vaginal dryness to boot.

Rheumatoid Arthritis

Problems with arousal, orgasm, and overall sexual satisfaction aren't all tied to decreased mobility or pain from this chronic inflammatory disorder, which is more common in women than men. Feeling depressed or anxious as a result of the disease can be tied to it as well.

Thyroid Disorders

One in eight women will develop a thyroid disorder, where their thyroid gland produces too much thyroid hormone, creates too little of the hormone, becomes enlarged, or some other concern arises. Thyroid disease, which may appear right after pregnancy or menopause, can decrease the amount of lubrication in your vagina, thus making sex uncomfortable.

THE 3 TYPES OF SEXUAL DYSFUNCTION IN WOMEN

Clinically speaking, here's how doctors categorize the different types of low libido. Know the terminology so you can have an informed conversation with your MD.

1. Pain Disorders

You're experiencing vaginismus (an involuntary tightening of the muscles around the vagina that causes discomfort with sex) or dyspareunia (a general term for persistent or recurrent pain before, during, or after intercourse). Your doctor has to do a thorough physical exam to figure out how to solve the problem, but know that the leading cause of dyspareunia is psychological.

2. Orgasmic Disorder

Either you can't have an orgasm at all (anorgasmic) or it takes a very long time to achieve one. Counseling, masturbation instruction, and a review of the medications you're taking have been shown to be helpful.

3. Arousal and Sexual Desire Disorder

The former is when you can't get wet enough to start or finish the act—and it's making you frustrated or causing problems with your relationship. A review of the medications you may be taking can often pinpoint the problem. The latter is when you're not interested in sex and you might even have an aversion to it—and it's making you frustrated or causing problems in your relationship.

BOOST YOUR SUPPLEMENTAL KNOWLEDGE, BOOST YOUR LIBIDO

When their libido flame is flickering low, I've seen women who are willing to try anything to get it at full force again. But I've also seen women who are more cautious and wary of options that require a prescription. Just in case you were wondering, there are plenty of natural alternatives on the market. Yes, herbal supplements are worth your time and your hard-earned money, according to my colleague, Tasneem "Dr. Taz" Bhatia, MD, an integrative health expert and the medical director at CentreSpring MD. Ready-to-go options like Zestra, a hormone-free topical blend of botanical oils and extracts, have been shown in studies to increase not only your desire but also your sexual satisfaction. If you're fine with a DIY approach, Dr. Taz has the following libido-lifters on her list: ginseng, maca, fenugreek, red clover, and arginine. But don't run to your health food store just yet. You need to work with your doctor to develop a plan for working supplements into your diet as part of a whole-body approach that evaluates your overall physical health, stress levels, hormones, nutrition, and gut health.

POINT OF V: HEED A DIFFERENT HOLY TRINITY

Successful women never stop pursuing their goals. They just keep chasing after them, only looking back to see what they've accomplished so far. If your sex drive isn't where you want it to be, then keep searching for the reason why you're not getting the ooh-ooh-ooh you deserve. Every woman's libido is a holy trinity of her mind, her body, and her soul.

When I say your mind, I mean that the fire in your Queen V is stoked by how you think and feel about your partner. Are they giving you your Vitamin S? When I talk about your body, that's everything physical. Do you know where your hot spots are? Have you shown your partner? And when I mention your soul, I'm shining a light on your spirit. If you don't love yourself—if you don't know how smart, beautiful, important, and worthy of love you are—how can you expect someone else to love you?

Despite the fact that we all have these three factors in play, your VP determines which are more important to you than others. My Sanctified Snatches, for example, might need more of their soul stoked than their body or mind. My Notorious V.A.G.s tend to need their partners to focus on their body more than their mind or soul. Figure out your balance and use it to keep your Queen V satisfied.

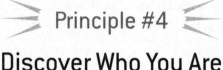

Principle #4

Discover Who You Are
in Bed—Every Day

WELCOME TO SPAGHETTI JUNCTION

In Germany, there's an 8,073-mile stretch of highway referred to as the Autobahn. For the most part, it has no official speed limit. You can drive as fast as you like on fairly straight freeways to get from city to city. I think for many men, getting sexually aroused is a lot like driving on the Autobahn. You can speed along at 120 miles per hour from point A (getting him excited) to point B (getting him orgasmic).

In Georgia, where I live, there's a complex intersection of highways called Spaghetti Junction. Its roads crisscross and circle each other from above and below. And there's definitely a speed limit. When it comes to sexual arousal, I think many women are a bit like Atlanta's Spaghetti Junction. Your partner has got to pay attention to the signs, they will definitely need to bring some patience, and they might get confused as you go from point A (getting excited) to point B (getting orgasmic). So I want to help you give your partner some solid directions from the passenger's seat.

In the last chapter, I got really honest with you about the emotional side of the sexual drive. Well, adjust your seat and buckle up, because in this chapter we are hitting the gas on the physical side of your sexual drive. Before you let your partner stick a key in the ignition and get on the road to orgasm, there are a few things I want you to do:

First, adjust your mirrors. So many of us are walking around with bad body image. We're feeling insecure about our weight, the size of our breasts, or any scars that we might have from pregnancy or surgery. Let's end it all. Right here. Right now. It's important to feel comfortable in your own skin before you share yourself with someone else. Those scars? They're battle trophies that show you came out stronger on the other side of something difficult. You're a badass! Those few extra pounds? They should never steal the joy of a good time in bed. While most of us continue to work on becoming happy, healthy, and wealthy, there are only a few perfectly proportioned supermodels. And they're not the only ones entitled to great sex. Low self-esteem could be a blind spot that sabotages your sex ride. Take a good look in the mirror and decide to love what you've got so you can let someone else love it too.

Next, eliminate distractions. Make sure the radio's tuned to your favorite station or your Spotify mix is playing so you don't have to fiddle with your sound system later. Put your cell phone away or at least flip it over so you don't see that news alert pop up. You want to focus on the road ahead.

Then, decide your destination. You probably haven't heard anyone say this before, but there are countless reasons for having sex and you should be clear, concise, and honest about what yours are. Do you need some tender, loving affection? Are you stressed as hell and trying to take the edge off? Do you want to get pregnant? Are you just trying to keep your partner happy? Is this an opportunity to broaden your sexual horizons by trying something new? Do you have a chance to "ride with" someone who is really hot and about to boost your self-esteem? Knowing what you want to get out of your sexual road trip can help ensure that you arrive at your destination faster and don't end up making a wrong turn. (Speaking of which, we'll be talking about preventing STIs and unplanned pregnancies in Principles #5, 6, and 7.) I want you to be able to skip any guilt trips and let yourself enjoy the scenery along the way.

Finally, be your own GPS. When your partner is trying to navigate your Spaghetti Junction, you're the best person to explain to him or her how to touch you here and stroke you there. No one knows your body better than you do. Here's the million-dollar orgasm question: What do you like?

HOW TO SET YOUR GPS FOR
SEXUAL SATISFACTION

"I've got a question, Dr. Jackie," one of my Mary Jane patients began during our appointment. "I'm into rimming but I want to make sure that when my husband switches to giving me oral sex there's no, you know, cross contamination." (For those of you who don't know, rimming is oral anal sex. Still confused? That's tongue in and around your back door.) She was right to be concerned about bacteria hitching a ride and causing her problems—even though she said her man uses mouthwash in between. (Using a dental dam would be cleaner.) But here's a surprise: I'm not telling you this story for a hygiene lesson on avoiding infections. I'm telling you this because it takes something different to turn on everyone's engine. As long as you're safe about it, vroom-vroom! Let your V be free.

This Mary Jane had figured out what she liked in bed and just wanted to make sure she could get it safely. (As I said: a dental dam could help them do that.) Finding what excites *you* is a little chemistry experiment I encourage you to do as often as possible, ladies. You have to know what you want if you expect to get it. It's not fair to ask your partner to guess whether they should be knocking on door number one, two, or three—and then what to do once it opens.

Right about now, I can hear my Notorious V.A.G.s and a lot of my Mary Janes saying to themselves, "I know exactly what I want." If so, congrats on being too blessed to be sexually stressed. But for my Virgin Marys, Sanctified Snatches, Coochie-Chondriacs, and some Mary Janes still on a road to discovery, you might need a few suggestions to help you help your partners. And that's what I'm here for.

1. **Do you.** Literally, get in touch with yourself. Yes, I'm suggesting sexual exploration. Everyone knows the top hot spots that are likely to excite them: lips, breasts, Queen V. But you have erogenous zones all over your body that deserve some exploration as well. What if stroking the edge of your ear is an epic-level turn-on? Ever take some time massaging the inside of your thigh to see how you'd react? When I asked my Instagram followers about the intimate things they like in bed they thought they'd never do, one respondent said, "Just touching! Touch is so important. On my body, on my face. Sheesh, my feet!" Finding those other tantalizing targets helps *your partner* be a better lover and *you* get better loving.

2. **Flip some pages.** I've got an important task for every Virgin Mary or Sanctified Snatch who didn't know what to say when a partner asked, "What's your fantasy?" Read a book. Whether it's a romance novel, the *Kama Sutra*, or some of the Zane chronicles, you're bound to come across some sexy situations you'd like to experience in real life. Now I have heard it said that there is nothing sexier than a man unloading a dishwasher or vacuuming the living room carpet without being asked. But remember, this chapter is about physical turn-ons, not emotional ones. Getting hot watching your man clean the shower is about emotional support. Getting hot thinking about your man pleasing you in the shower is what I'm talking about right here.

3. **Treat yourself.** If you're too embarrassed to walk into an adult toy store, think about browsing around online. From blindfolds and nurse's outfits to nipple toys and butt plugs, you're sure to be surprised by something that could spark your arousal. If you're not sure where your pleasure points are, vibrators and dildos can help. I should mention that there are several touchpoints inside your Queen V that can make you hit the ceiling. Check out Principle #8 on sex toys for ways to explore those spots solo and with your partner.

4. **Take a peek at an erotic movie.** Let's be clear: I'm not advocating

pornography. But there are women who have found their sexual Shangri-La by watching steamy movies.

5. **Have bold experiences.** Your first time having sex is a little like your first time driving a car. You don't know where to put your hands, you're not sure what direction to look in, and you can't wait to rev that engine! Here's the thing though: you have no idea what that car can do from your first time taking it out. The same is true of your body. None of us get a PhD in carnal knowledge after a single sack session. It's going to take a lot more sexual encounters to figure out what you like in bed. You and your partner might try role-playing, different positions, and other locations to tap into your turn-ons. "I like finding secret places to be intimate," one of my Instagram followers revealed to me.

It doesn't take multiple partners to have bold experiences—but some of us will uncover them that way. "I never liked cunnilingus," another Instagram follower admitted. "But with the right person it's amazing." Another told me that she never thought she'd be into giving a man oral sex, but she is now. Well, sometimes: "I've learned that the more selfless a man is in the bedroom, the more I open up to it."

The awkward but amazing sex you had with your college boyfriend or girlfriend won't be the same as the clandestine and quick sex you have with the coworker you're dating at your first job. Or the person who comes after that. Don't forget that a new partner can bring out a new VP in you as well. So don't be surprised if you feel yourself shifting from a Virgin Mary to a Sanctified Snatch or from a Mary Jane to a Notorious V.A.G. with different partners. In fact, why not enjoy it?

UNCOVER YOUR QUEEN V'S SUPERPOWERS

Part of discovering *who* you are in bed is discovering *what* you can do in bed. Your Queen V is capable of so much more than just giving you one satisfying, toe-curling orgasm. Her only kryptonite would be an ingness to explore all these pleasurable possibilities.

Edging. Up the ante on your orgasm exponentially with this technique of getting to the brink of orgasm, then backing off for several seconds and then approaching the edge again. You can do this on your own (while self-exploring) or with a partner (so long as you communicate how close you are to coming). It may take some practice to get it right. You don't want to lose your climax entirely by waiting too long or repeating the on-again-off-again method too many times. But those who have mastered this move that delays orgasm say it leads to off-the-charts, full-body climax in the end. If you've got some free time on your hands, it might be worth a go.

Orgasms (single, sequential multiple, serial multiple, and blended). Imagine orgasms as a sort of sexual fireworks celebration. Sometimes just one firework gets shot into the air, it explodes in a single big boom, and that's more than enough to rock your world. That's a single orgasm. Other times you've got a few fireworks in your back pocket. You send one up and it goes off. Then you take a break for a minute and then light another and it goes off. And so on. Those are sequential multiple orgasms. You might think your clitoris is too sensitive for stimulation immediately after climaxing, but give it a few seconds and check in. You'd be surprised.

Next, imagine you've got one firework that explodes into a series of rapid-fire bursts. Boom-boom-boom-boom-boom! That's what we call serial multiple orgasms. Finally, let's say you lit two fireworks at the same time and sent them into the air. Let's imagine that's you getting clitoral stimulation to orgasm and, say, anal stimulation to orgasm as well. (But really, any two—or more—erogenous orgasm zones will do.) That would be a blended orgasm. We're all built differently, so not everyone will be able to or want to achieve every type of orgasm. But wouldn't it be fun to try a few?

Pompoir. Before I heard the word pompoir, I just heard stories of women who could clench their pelvic floor muscles so tightly their man's penis couldn't move an inch. Yes, honey. I'm talking about control. Did you hear me? I keep telling you all that your Queen V is ready to rule. Maybe you've heard it called the Singapore Kiss, the Kabazza, or Milking the Penis. They're all just different terms for the same thing: an ancient sexual technique in which you use your vaginal muscles to push, pull, lock down on, twist, and do even more to your man's penis for an incredible orgasm. He literally doesn't have to move at all. You put in all the effort, normally from a girl-on-top position.

Squirting. Ever wonder what it feels like for men when they ejaculate? Some women say they don't have to wonder. They can feel the exact same thing themselves. Yes, you read that right. Female ejaculation is a thing. A hotly debated thing. There are experts who say the Skene's gland of the urethra (think of it as the female prostate gland) can involuntarily dribble or gush a whitish fluid during sex. Others say there's nothing to see here. Move along. This is basically urban legend or simply urine leaking out. I'm always going to be honest with you ladies, so I'll tell you that most of my patients who squirt tell me that it doesn't smell like urine. None of them have ever complained of it hurting, but they do tell me that it's an amazing release.

While it might sound incredible, squirting can interfere with your sex life. When one patient of mine told me about her ability to squirt, I said, "Man, that must be some good sex." She shook her head: "I feel like I'm peeing in the bed and my husband is over it," she said. If you've got a Queen V that can erupt like Mount St. Helens, you've got to inform your partner, assure them that it's completely normal, and, of course, have a towel handy in bed. But trying to prevent yourself from squirting might also prevent you from experiencing sexual pleasure.

ASKING FOR WHAT YOU WANT
BETWEEN THE SHEETS

Next to answering your phone during sex (hello? Rude) and not recip-
rocating (ladies, don't kneel for it), there's nothing worse than a sexual
partner who's in the wrong place at the right time. A plus-size Mary Jane
once confided in me that her boyfriend fit this description perfectly. He
thought he was penetrating her, but he was just thrusting into the folds
of her thighs. He just knew he was really doing something down there,
but she wasn't getting "done" at all—just knocking his own socks off.
And MJ couldn't bring herself to tell him for fear of hurting his feelings.
Ladies, if your man's orgasm is off the Richter Scale, then your orgasm
better be out-of-this-world seismic activity too. Don't settle for steady
ground.

To get there, you need to start talking. During pillow talk, I would
tease my husband by pretending to hold up a scorecard like an Olympic figure skating judge and saying, "That was a five." Or "Perfect ten!"
You don't have to pull out placards, but if you're not satisfied, you should
offer some gentle honesty and some firm coaching. Maybe your boyfriend
couldn't find your clitoris with the help of Siri, Alexa, and Google combined. Maybe your wife thinks foreplay is a foreign word. Maybe your
husband is going at you like a defective jackhammer. Whatever the case,
don't fake it until he or she makes it. Again, your anticlimactic issue isn't
libido. It's learning. Your partner wants the neighbors across the hall (hey,
down the block too) to know they get the job done. They just need a few
pointers from you to get there.

By now, I've explained the who (your partner) and the what (your
desires in bed). Now it's time for the rest of the five Ws (and an H).

When. Telling someone you're into spanking may not go over well
on the first or second date. (Isn't that the truth?) Wait until
you're at a place in your relationship where there's a sense of trust

and security. While you can give quick feedback when you're in bed ("Move over here, baby" or "A little to the left"), it's best to make sure longer conversations ("Would you ever consider anal?") don't happen right before or right after sex. One will put a lot of pressure on your partner. The other is a point in time when you're feeling incredibly vulnerable and rejection could feel terrible.

Where. Depends on your level of sexual emotional intelligence. Usually outside the bedroom is best. Maybe when you're watching a movie in the living room or strolling through one of those sex shops I mentioned above. But some couples work it into their pillow talk just fine.

Why. Come on now. You know why. Get all the ooh-ooh-ooh you deserve, girl!

How. It's been said that 55 percent of communication is body language. That means you don't even have to talk during sex to get some of what you want. If he needs a road map to find your G-spot, just take the wheel (or his hand) and show him. Nudge his lips over here, turn your body in another direction over there, and get what you want.

If actions aren't quite speaking louder than words, but you're nervous about piping up, consider giving him feedback in just one word. Think "softer," "here," "harder," "yes," "ouch." Be sure to use your soft and seductive porn voice. You know what I'm talking about.

Once you're outside the bedroom, that's when things can really get interesting. Let all that self-exploration research that you've been doing finally pay off. Tell him or her about something sexy you saw in a movie or read in a book, then ask if they'd be willing to try it. If you need to discourage some behavior, remember to be gentle. I had a patient whose boyfriend kept blowing in her ear during sex. "He thinks I like it but it drives me insane," she said. "I just want to scream." Before you do, try a calmer approach. Be kind but be clear about what turns you on and what doesn't quite do it for you. You'll get more of what you like and less of what's blowing out your sexual flame.

WHEN YOU WOULD DO ANYTHING FOR LOVE—BUT YOU WON'T DO *THAT*

You always hear people say, "Don't knock it until you've tried it." I don't know if that's true. When you're grown, you know your limits. There's no need to deny them. If you're not in the least bit curious about a threesome or S&M—and your partner is—it's important to be up-front and clear with them about it. You can simply say, "I just don't feel comfortable doing that." Remember, sex isn't just about one person. It's about everyone involved in the act.

Now, you may find yourself in a situation where you tried something, didn't like it, but you are willing do it for your partner. You need to be vocal about that too. I know it's not the most feminist thing for me to say, but it happens in relationships. You can tell your partner, "I'm not really into oral sex, but I know you enjoy it. I won't do this every night, but I will once in a while." Oh, and real talk: you should expect the same type of compromise from your partner as well.

THE SPECIALIST'S CORNER: SEX THERAPY, PART 2

Chances are your high school sex ed class didn't teach you how to ask your partner if they're into a little BDSM. (By the way, that's bondage and discipline, dominance and submission, sadism and masochism.) That's what I'm here for. In the previous chapter, I asked Tiffanie Davis Henry, PhD, a certified sex therapist and relationship expert in Atlanta, Georgia, to give us her expert insight into libido. In our second "V" Q&A on getting the loving you want, she explains the worst thing you can ever do in bed, her sandwich method for having it your way romantically, and the sex list every woman should make for herself.

Dr. Jackie: You once told me a great question women should ask *themselves* before asking *their partner* for something sexual in bed.

> **Dr. Tiffanie:** Yes: ask yourself, "What is your expectation of this relationship?" If it's just someone you want to have sex with, then it's super important that you put those sexual requests out there. But if this is someone you want to marry or have kids with, hold on. You might put your needs in a hierarchy. The fact that he or she is a good provider, for example, might be more important than him or her not wanting to get into anal play with you.

Dr. Jackie: I asked my Instagram followers why they don't ask for what they want in bed and so many women told me they were too embarrassed or worried to speak up. What's that about?

> **Dr. Tiffanie:** It doesn't surprise me that some people aren't 100 percent comfortable bringing up their preferences. Not too long ago we were in the age of *Fifty Shades of Grey* where women were thinking, "Maybe anal beads aren't such a weird thing!" The book and the movie normalized what was once thought of to be kinkier sex and more and more women became willing to explore. Now we've walked it back a bit as we've become more empowered about our likes and dislikes; wanting sex but on our terms. It's an interesting 180 that we've done. At the end of the day, much of what we tend to be afraid of is rejection. Many of us resist advocating for what we want sexually or fear our partners will deny us or reject us because of our desires. Rather than face rejection, many women remain silent.

Dr. Jackie: So are there some women just following their partner's lead in bed, like when you're dancing?

> **Dr. Tiffanie:** Yes. In fact, the worst thing you can ever do is be a pillow princess in bed. Just lie back and let your partner do whatever. No quid pro quo. It's not always girls who do that either. Sometimes it's guys. I know a guy who has become a very lazy lover because he's so attractive and girls would do anything for him. Another thing: sometimes we fall into routines. There are plenty of older couples who have sex in the same way every time: a few minutes of finger play, a few minutes of oral sex, a few minutes of vaginal sex, climax, then they roll over and go to sleep. You being afraid to ask for something may not be a *them* problem. It may be a *you* problem. Maybe you're getting complacent.

Dr. Jackie: Okay, so let's get some needs met. If you're in a relationship, you can just suggest something new you'd like to try. But what if you want to stop your partner from doing something that's already been happening?

> **Dr. Tiffanie:** I always recommend the sandwich method: give them something positive you like, something to improve upon, and then another positive. So say, "I really love it when you kiss my neck like that. It makes me scream every time. But when you're fingering me, if you could just trim your nails a bit, it kinda scratched me a little last time. But when you touch me there, it makes me so excited."

Dr. Jackie: Love it! I call that the Oreo! Why does it work?

> **Dr. Tiffanie:** If you start out with "Your nails are a mess!" Then all they hear is what they did wrong. Especially with guys, their egos are much more fragile than we realize. You have to

buffer the bad with compliments and praise so they get the
message.

**Dr. Jackie: How do you suggest handling sexual requests that you don't
want to try?**

> **Dr. Tiffanie:** Don't shame your partner. Instead be curious. Balance
> that part of you that's totally turned off by it with the part that
> is inquisitive. Let's say your partner wants to try anal sex. You
> could tell them, "You know I've never tried that before. Have
> you? Tell me about it." Or try, "Hmm, I'm really scared of that.
> I heard the anus doesn't have any lubrication. What makes you
> want to experience that?" If you're never going to go there, just
> be gentle but honest. You could say, "That's not something I
> think I'd ever do." Or try, "I love you, but I'm not interested in
> that."

**Dr. Jackie: What if your partner is really, really into something and
you're having trouble turning them down?**

> **Dr. Tiffanie:** I like to ask my patients to make "Always, Sometimes,
> and Never" lists. On the Always list, you write down acts
> you're always down for in bed. On the Sometimes list, put the
> acts that aren't your thing, but you'll do them sometimes to
> please the other person or switch things up. Never is "Please
> don't ever ask me to do that." You'd be amazed how writing
> this out—either for yourself or with your partner—helps
> things in the bedroom. When you make the list with a partner,
> you realize that everyone has their hang-ups. It becomes
> unreasonable to ask someone to do something they say they
> "never" want to do when you have things you "never" want
> to do on your list too. But you also get to see what's on their
> Always and Sometimes lists. Your partner may never want to
> do X, but will always and sometimes do Y and Z. So there

may be a compromise that makes everyone happy. Maybe you'd never be interested in a threesome, but sometimes you will watch same-sex porn while being intimate with your partner instead. That could get everyone's needs met without compromising anyone.

Dr. Jackie: What's the one thing everyone needs to remember about boldly, kindly, and clearly asking for what they want in bed?

Dr. Tiffanie: This is going to sound surprising, but in a sermon the other day, my pastor said, "You have not because you ask not." He wasn't talking about sexual relationships, but it does apply. You can't be mad about what you don't have in your relationship if you haven't articulated what your needs are. Men are notorious for not being able to read our minds. They don't have that gift. So if you're in a heterosexual relationship, it's not fair to keep them guessing or grasping at straws. Most men want you to be pleased and happy during sex. They want you to tell your girlfriends about what an amazing job they do. At the end of the night, if you're not getting what you want in bed and you haven't articulated it, don't be mad at anyone except yourself.

POINT OF V: GET SEXUALLY STRATEGIC

People choose to have sex for two reasons and two reasons alone: procreation and recreation. Both paths should involve a fair amount of planning, but usually only one does. When women are focused on procreation, they track their cycles to figure out when they're going to ovulate and stock their medicine cabinets with pregnancy tests. When women are focused on recreation, they're not nearly as tactical. That's a shame because men could really use some help and you could be having a much better boot-knocking experience.

Remember, there is no finish line when it comes to carnal pleasure.

Every time I read the Bible I discover something different. It's the same thing with sex. You can always find something new and different that you hadn't explored before if you keep an open mind. Get to know what you like, get comfortable asking for it, and get goal-oriented between the sheets. It's been said that it's not the destination, it's the journey. But why not enjoy both?

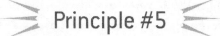

Principle #5

Get as Down and Dirty as You Want—But Remember This

THE POPE OF YOUR VAGINA

Urinary tract infections are one of the most painful conditions to deal with, and at one point, I had a Virgin Mary patient who got them like clockwork. She sat on the edge of the pink exam table staring at a painting on the wall so she didn't have to look directly at me. "I always notice this problem after I . . . *you know*," she said in a quiet, shy voice. No, I didn't know. In fact, it took a lot of gentle probing to try to pull the answer out of her. Eventually I guessed it: "After you masturbate?" I asked her. "Yeah," she said, almost in a whisper. To this day, I don't know what she was masturbating with that kept giving her UTIs. *A cucumber? A showerhead? A hairbrush handle?* Whatever it was, she didn't want to talk about it. And I couldn't pry it out of her—which is a problem.

I preach the gospel of caring for your V, I offer counsel to people going through tough times, and I listen to (sexual) confessions on a daily basis, so you might call me the Pope of your V. I'm not here to judge you. I'm here to use the information you give me to treat you. So it's absolutely critical that you don't hold back details about what you're doing behind closed doors. By hearing all the, ahem, ins and outs of your sexcapades, I can offer you better advice. You should always reveal to your doctor anything new (or anyone new) that you've introduced to your vagina whether you bought it in a store or brought him home from a bar. Had my Virgin Mary patient given me more details, I might have realized that she just needed some advice on how to clean dirt off produce.

One big reason I think patients withhold information is that they think what they're doing is shameful (say, having a threesome . . . or a foursome) or strange (say, foot sex or fisting). I assure you: you're not making history with your sexual exploits. Google whatever you're doing and you'll see someone else has already done it. While joining the mile-high club. In first class.

Everyone's entitled to get as down and dirty as they want, but I need you to come clean when you walk into my confession booth of an exam room. I also need you to follow this advice for protecting your Queen V from vaginal infections, STIs, or worse in any sexy situation. No Hail Marys necessary.

HOW TO PROTECT YOUR QUEEN V IN ANY SEXY SITUATION

Sexy Situation #1: Pouring *Anything* on Your Partner (or Yourself)

Coconut oil. Chocolate syrup. Massage oil. Honey. You name it, I've heard of people bringing it to bed. If it comes in a bottle and it's going in your vagina, let it be a water-based lubricant. Period. Special formulations like Astroglide and Sliquid won't alter the pH of your Queen V or change the permeability of a condom. Other lubes, lotions, and potions can end up being a disaster. If you're giving your partner a sexy massage with baby oil or body lotion, don't rub or tug anything that will enter or approach your vagina (without wiping it off) unless you want a vaginal infection. Intent on adding natural oils like coconut and olive to sex play? Sorry, leave them in the kitchen instead of on a path of destruction against a latex condom. (It's all right for polyurethane though.) I've heard of patients using everything from petroleum jelly (sure, it seems harmless but could give you bacterial vaginosis) to whipped cream (sexy, but combined with penetration it can bake up some yeast).

Speaking of pouring things on, it's also important to share a few words about safety around bringing candle wax into the bedroom. Some people like a little pain mixed in with their pleasure—whether you're giving or receiving a hot wax treatment—but your Queen V's skin is very thin. It wasn't designed to tolerate 145 degrees of foreplay (yes, that's how hot candle wax can get). Sometimes, although you're careful, accidents can happen. "I was having a little kinky sex," one patient told me when she came in with first-degree burns. "He poured some hot wax up here, but it rolled down there pretty quickly and . . . Ooh!" Unfortunately, there's not much you can do after the fact besides using cortisone cream (externally) for a bit of a cooling sensation and just waiting for your skin to heal. If it's more than a first-degree burn, you may want to see your OB-GYN to eliminate any risk of infection. In addition to being careful about where you pour the wax, be sure to avoid a splash effect. (The higher you start the drip, the more time it has to cool on its way down—but too far leads to splashing.) Finally, if you do decide to toy with a taper or play with a votive near your privates—I know some of you are tough as nails and into S&M—remember that many candles have perfumes, dyes, and other additives that your Queen V may react to.

I'll say a final word about a last-ditch lubricant a lot of people use: saliva. Just remember that saliva can pass along sexually transmitted infections as well. It's also not as slippery as anything you'd buy in a store, so you could still have some uncomfortable friction. Ouch!

Sexy Situation #2: Ménage à Moi

As the song goes, learning to love yourself is the greatest love of all. It's the absolute ultimate in self-care—unless you do yourself wrong. Imagine that your Queen V is sitting on her throne holding court. The visitors who walk down that red carpet to meet with her come bearing extraordinary gifts to impress her. Make sure you do the same. That means no rubbing up against a pillowcase covered in hair product, no soaping up and then aiming the showerhead between your legs, and no twerking up against sex toys you haven't gotten around to cleaning. Make sure your party of one stays all fun and safe.

Sexy Situation #3: Getting It On with Sex Toys

From sculpted stainless steel to cyberskin, which offers a real skin feel, sex toys are here to please us. But they deserve a little tender loving care in return. That's why it's important that you (if you're flying solo) or your partner (if you're getting it on with somebody else) clean them after each and every use. What's so bad about a dirty sex toy? Especially if you're the only one using it? Not cleaning them thoroughly can leave bacteria growing on them that you'd be exposed to on your next use and increase your risk of getting an infection. When you're sharing sex toys, know that if the other person who used them has a sexually transmitted infection, you could get it too. Finally, avoid passing your toy from one orifice (say, your anus) to another (like your vagina). Letting bacteria hitch a ride from your back door to your Queen V could result in a serious infection.

Because sex toys are made of various porous and nonporous materials both with and without motors, they all need to be cleaned in different ways. Toys made of silicone that are motorized, for example, can be cleaned with a gentle soap and water, whereas silicone toys that aren't motorized can be placed in boiling water or run through the dishwasher (without detergent) for a deep clean. Rubber toys are worth rolling a condom onto for easier cleanup, while cyberskin ones usually only require warm water. To avoid destroying the material your orgasmic investment is made of, your best bet is to read the cleaning instructions that came with your toy or search for them online if you don't have the packaging anymore. Then dry it with a clean paper towel and store it in the pouch it came with to keep it safe from other elements. One last word of caution: do not use silicone- or oil-based lube with your silicone sex toys—it breaks down their material.

Curious about using other household items as sex toys (which is a no-no in my book) or want more cleaning tips? Check out Principle #8: Know When to Leave Sex Toys to the Professionals.

Sexy Situation #4: Receiving or Giving Oral Sex

There are three things you need to remember whether your partner is "dining at the Y" or you're going down on them. First, protection. Second, protection. And third, this is really important and you won't see it coming: protection. Barrier methods of protection, like a dental dam, can protect you from diseases if you use them consistently and properly. (I know, few people use them. But they can keep you safe.) You'll want to choose oral sex protection that is latex, polyurethane, or polyisoprene—but not lambskin.

I know this might sound stuffy and not everyone is on board, but I've seen the consequences of not using protection with oral sex. Diseases like herpes, human papillomavirus (HPV), gonorrhea, and syphilis not only impact genitalia but can also infect your mouth, throat, and anus.

One more word of caution before your partner prepares for a box lunch: yeast infections can also be transmitted via oral sex. If the person you're getting hot and bothered with has thrush in their mouth (or even their throat, where it would be hard for you to see), they can pass it along to you when they head downtown. So a little protection goes a long way.

Having oral anal sex (also known as analingus or rimming)? See Sexy Situation #7.

Sexy Situation #5: Penetration

Years ago, a college student came to see me in tears because of bladder pain. She thought she might have a urinary tract infection at best and at worst some tumor or something. What she never imagined was that the pain was due to a herpes outbreak happening inside her bladder. (Yes, you read that right.) She was in a long-term relationship with a young man who had the disease—but he was too embarrassed to tell her, and she never noticed him having an outbreak. (It's also worth mentioning that there can be asymptomatic viral shedding leading to the transmission of herpes.) When they committed to not seeing other people, they decided to have unprotected sex. And, well, you know how that story ended in my office.

It's never easy to tell someone that you have a sexually transmitted infection. But it's definitely essential before things get physical between you. Until you both get tested, you can protect yourself from unpleasant surprises by using latex, polyurethane, or polyisoprene condoms for penetrative sex. Cover up and keep the party going.

Sexy Situation #6: Scheduling a Sexathon

Release the balloons, signal the band, and cue the applause. Congratulations, girl! If you're lucky enough to have a partner who wants to give it to you all day long—or all weekend long—put down this book for a second, pick up your phone, and let them know they're your hero. Seriously. I'll wait.

Now back to your Queen V: just like marathoners who stock up on chafing lotions and Gatorade before race day, you need to stock up on some supplies before you lock the doors, leave the world behind, and have nonstop sex. You could get parched. Everywhere. So make sure you have plenty of water to drink and lube to rub on. (Vaginal tearing is a real concern and can result from too much friction during sex or being too dry.) While some couples have a sexfest for fun, others do it to try to get pregnant. If baby-making is your goal, be sure to choose a lube that says it's sperm-friendly on the label. These don't contain ingredients like glycerin that can harm sperm. They also try to mimic the pH of your vagina for a more hospitable environment.

Regardless of your bumping and grinding goals, when you're doing "missionary work" or joining the "cow girl" hall of fame or counting to "69," you should pee a few minutes before and after sex. It will help you avoid getting "honeymoon cystitis"—that's just a much prettier name for a urinary infection as a result of a whole lot of action. This is especially important for women who are prone to infections. Back in the day, I used to give patients a prescription for an antibiotic if they told me they were headed out of the country for their honeymoon. Nothing puts a damper on a weekend in paradise like getting an infection and having to find a doctor in an unfamiliar land.

Sexy Situation #7: Enjoying Anal Sex

"I swear it's the most intense orgasm. Ever," said one of my Notorious V.A.G. patients when she was telling me about letting her man get to "fifth base." In my experience, most women have either a love or a hate relationship with anal sex. The concentration of nerve endings around the entrance to your anus can certainly make it enjoyable (ouch, ooh, oh!). In fact, orgasms are a gloriously frequent occurrence for women who have anal sex. One survey found that while about 66 percent of women who had recently had vaginal sex had orgasms, a whopping 94 percent of women who had recently had anal sex had orgasms. (Of course, anal probably wasn't the only thing that happened while they were going at it.)

Then comes the hate part. Unlike your vagina, the anal canal doesn't self-lubricate. So if you're planning to join the (approximately) one in three women who have let their partner slip in the back door, you've got to bring your own lube to the party (or somebody should). Anything else could be painful. Silicone lube is perfect for anal sex because it's thicker and a bit more slippery. Having a patient partner and talking frequently during your anal adventures makes all the difference as well. Entry into what is usually an exit orifice can be . . . intense. You have to communicate clearly with your partner about what feels good and what doesn't, when to stop, and if it's all right to start again.

All the preventive measures for penetrative sex still apply. The inner lining of the anal canal (the mucosa) is easier to tear than the lining of the vagina, so you'll be at increased risk of getting an STI. Make sure that you use a latex, polyurethane, or polyisoprene condom to protect yourself from sexually transmitted infections. Some experts recommend "extra strong" and already lubricated condoms for backdoor adventures. If you switch from anal to vaginal, you must make sure that your partner uses a new condom, cleans their penis, or cleans the sex toy they're using before switching to a new location. If not, you could wind up with bacterial vaginosis, a yeast infection, or a urinary tract infection.

A word about oral anal sex. Remember the Mary Jane patient I told you about who asked me about the risks of switching from oral anal sex to oral vaginal in terms of spreading bacteria? She and her husband liked to switch from one to the other with their tongues. Here's the deal: it poses the exact same risk of spreading bacteria that going from penetrative anal to penetrative vaginal does. So use a new dental dam for each sex act to be safe.

Sexy Situation #8: Toeing and Footplay

Peep-toe shoes. Pretty pedicures. Sexy sandals. Toes are a turn-on for a lot of people. And if you're introducing them to your Queen V, you've got to be careful. Case in point: during my residency, there was a woman who came in every two weeks with recurrent yeast infections. This went on for four months. I kept gently asking her: "Is there anything going in your vagina that you aren't telling me about?" Finally, she told me that her husband likes to insert his toes into her vagina. Well, once we got his athlete's foot cured, my patient stopped getting yeast infections.

If you're into feet—and they're into you—just make sure that they're clean and fungus-free so you avoid yeast infections. It's best to ask your partner if they've had jock itch between their toes. Have they had any itching or burning sensations in between their toes or on their soles? But you can also look for any redness, dryness, peeling skin, or rashes on their feet. Once you're sure they're fungus-free, there's no better time for a pedicure to make sure your partner doesn't have long, sharp, or jagged nails that could cut your delicate vaginal skin (yes, ow!).

Sexy Situation #9: Fingering and Fisting

A few words to the wise when it comes to letting someone insert their fingers, their fist, or more into your vagina: Be careful. Be comfortable with it. And be sure it's not painful.

I'm hoping that your partner has done their homework when it comes to these practices, because there's an art to them. It's not just about poking or punching a woman's vagina. Women who rave about fingering are on the receiving end of a hand that knows how to stimulate her G-spot, tantalize the walls of her vagina, and put just the right amount of pressure on her clitoris. Women who deeply enjoy fisting often talk about the feeling of "fullness" that it gives them. But these moves take patience and practice.

Make sure your partner goes slow when entering *and* exiting your Queen V. They should also have nails that are short, manicured, and preferably polish-free. Finally, use plenty of lube—without numbing agents. Lubes with numbing agents can make you less aware of how much pain you might be in. You can still pass along yeast infections, bacterial vaginosis, and sexually transmitted infections via your hands. (And, real talk: just think about everything else your bare hands have picked up, scratched, rubbed on, brushed against, or held on to in the past twenty-four hours. They're a pretty big buffet of bacteria.) No time to make sure your partner's hands and nails are clean before they slide inside you? Skip the clean routine by using a latex glove or mitten. Let your fingers do some clicking around any sex toy site and you'll find ones specially made for fisting.

Sexy Situation #10: Threesomes, Orgies, and Overlapping Partners

Occasionally patients tell me something purely for shock value (or so I think). They want to make sure I won't peer down my glasses at them. Trust me, I'm not judgy, but I haven't seen it all. Still, I didn't bat an eyelash when a Notorious V.A.G. came in for an appointment and told me, "You know, Dr. Jackie, sometimes my man and I have a third person in the bed." I've got patients who are swingers. I've also seen patients who are down with larger sex parties and, of course, Queen Vs who can't decide between different partners, so they're enjoying both at the same time.

I encourage all my patients to use condoms if they're engaging in sex with more than one person—and to use a fresh condom for each partner. It's not only to protect themselves from sexually transmitted infections but also to help prevent bacterial vaginosis. While there's no medical literature to support it, doctors have a theory that mixing vaginal flora (say, by allowing a man who has stuck his penis inside another woman to then roll over in bed and do the same to you without using or switching condoms) can lead to BV. Every woman's vaginal flora is unique to her. So when we're exposed to other types of flora, it can throw off our balance. Honey, it was never meant to mix both worlds at the same time.

Now's a good place to bring up the dreaded C-word . . . Cheating. It's worth mentioning that you can find yourself getting an STI or bacterial vaginosis if your partner is dibbling and dabbling in different floras. It's also possible if you're the one doing the dibbling and dabbling. One of my Mary Jane patients had romances going on with a husband and a boyfriend in another state. "This doesn't make me a bad person," she'd tell me when she ended up in my office with recurrent BV after a trip out of town. "It's just someone I've had in my life that I can't let go." Sadly, she'd complain to her husband that *he* was the problem—in an attempt to cover her tracks. I don't tell people how to behave in their marriage, but I'm very vocal when it comes to how you treat your Queen V. If you're spreading yourself around, use protection. Period.

Sexy Situation #11: Rough Play and Bondage

After slowly walking into my office and carefully easing herself onto the exam room table, a patient said to me, "I think we tore something." Guess what? She had—and she was in excruciating vaginal pain. The night before, she and her man were having very vigorous cowgirl sex (that's woman on top, for those who haven't had the pleasure). I imagine she may have been bouncing more enthusiastically than she realized. Or perhaps he had his hands on her waist and pulled her down onto him more forcefully that he realized. Either way, the heat of passion led to a very hard penis tearing the wall of her vagina. I could barely get the speculum inside to see the split—which I sewed up later.

Ladies, just like us, the vagina is very forgiving. You can do a lot of things to her (insult her by giving her an infection, push her past her limits while pushing out a baby) and she'll come back to you stronger than ever. But that's not free rein to try her patience. No matter what you decide to do behind closed doors, make sure you have a conversation with your partner beforehand. Are you planning on some nail clawing, biting, or hair pulling? Ask permission outside the bedroom first—especially if you think you'll be yanking on a weave. Excited by a little choking, spanking, or heavier S&M? Get any shade of grey going that you please, but make sure you decide on a safe word so nothing goes too far. No one wants to meet their maker while having an orgasm. If you ever feel uncomfortable during sex, you simply must speak up.

7 TIMES TO GET TESTED FOR A SEXUALLY TRANSMITTED INFECTION

It's not fair, it's not your fault, but it's a fact: if you're sexually active, you're probably going to get some type of an infection at some point in your life. I can feel my Virgin Marys and Sanctified Snatches shaking their heads back and forth, but the numbers don't lie. Eighty percent of sexually active people have been infected with some strain of HPV (the STI that can cause genital warts and cervical cancer) in their lifetimes. No matter what you contract, you should never ignore it, you should confirm it with your doctor, and you must tell your partner (or partners) about it. We'll get to talking to your partner later in this chapter. In the meantime, let's address the seven occasions (yes, seven) that sexually active women should get tested for STIs.

1. Your Annual Exam

Some of my married patients will pass on this option because they trust that their partners aren't stepping out. I want you to trust your intuition more. Ladies, if your first gut reaction is to say yes to the test, then say yes. You can never, ever be 100 percent sure about something like that. Plus, many infections like chlamydia and HSV can be silent. That means that you may not have any signs of exposure (like discharge or bumps), but it could still be wreaking havoc on your reproductive system. It could also lead to scarring or create cancerous cells on your sexual organs. So it's best to err on the side of caution. It's covered by most insurance providers and it's good for your Queen V.

2. You Noticed Something

You felt a few bumps down there while in the shower? You saw a green-ish discharge in your bikini briefs? You picked up on an unusual smell? Whenever your vagina behaves, looks, or smells different from what you expect, it may be time to make an appointment with your MD to find out what's going on. The sooner the better. It's better for me to look at, for example, an active outbreak of herpes rather than one that happened three weeks ago.

3. You Had Unprotected Sex

Oops! You got swept off your feet, it was the heat of the moment, you didn't have a condom handy, and in that second you really didn't care one bit. Or perhaps nothing gets you hotter than anonymous sex. Or, and I'm so sorry if this is the case, maybe it was a much scarier situation where you were violated and forced into intercourse. Either way, testing can put your mind at ease about what you were exposed to through unprotected sex. It can take from several days to several months for your body to express signs of different types of STIs. So call your doctor and schedule an appointment immediately and refrain from unprotected sex in the meantime—but you'll have to wait. It's great to establish a baseline of no previous STIs. If you have a negative STI test a few days after sex and then three weeks later your STI test is positive, you probably got it from that person.

4. You Want to Have Unprotected Sex

Before you and your partner kick condoms to the curb, take the time to make sure you are both free from sexually transmitted infections. You deserve that and so does your partner.

5. Your Partner Tells You They Had Unprotected Sex

They tell you they cheated. You're seeing red. After the police leave (just kidding . . . kind of) you've got to look out for yourself—because they sure weren't looking out for you. Your newfound knowledge gives you an opportunity to protect your Queen V. Don't be embarrassed. Be her best advocate. Pick up the phone and make an appointment with your doctor.

6. Your Partner Has a Chronic Sexually Transmitted Infection

Getting a long-term STI like herpes, HIV, or hepatitis B or C doesn't mean you'll never get married, no one will ever love you, or you won't ever have sex again. Your love story isn't over if you have one of these diseases—and your love story doesn't have to be over if a potential partner tells you they have one of these diseases. It's possible to protect yourself from contracting the infection or transmitting it. As part of the precautions you take, you'll want to talk to your doctor about getting tested more frequently.

7. You're Trying to Get Pregnant or You Are Pregnant

Before you begin your baby quest, it's best to confirm that you don't have a sexually transmitted infection. A silent STI could delay your ability to get pregnant or decide how you'll be able to give birth. If you weren't able to check before conceiving, you'll definitely want to check once you find out you're pregnant.

COMMON INFECTIONS (AND HOW TO TREAT THEM)

When it comes to infections, the most important thing is to recognize that something isn't right in your body. Then you need to confirm the diagnosis with your doctor and eliminate your risk factors. It's as simple as that. Ignoring active infections (or not getting tested for asymptomatic ones so they go untreated) can lead to conditions like Pelvic Inflammatory Disease (PID). This condition can damage your reproductive organs and lower your fertility. And where there's one infection, sometimes there are more. So what are the conditions you should be on the lookout for? The most common ones are below:

Yeast Infection

What it is: Up to 75 percent of women will experience this fungal infection in their lifetime. It can cause vaginal itching, a burning sensation, and a discharge that may look like cottage cheese or chunks of wet toilet tissue.

Sometimes confused with: Bacterial vaginosis. They both cause a whitish discharge. I've also noticed that many women would rather tell me they have a yeast infection as opposed to saying they think they have BV. The latter sounds like a sexually transmitted infection they might be ashamed of. The former is something women are more comfortable saying they have because you can get it simply from wearing a bathing suit too long. (By the way, neither of them is a sexually transmitted infection.)

How to tell the difference: When examining yourself, see if the discharge has a scent. Yeast infections are usually odorless while bacterial vaginosis has a fishy smell. Also, don't be afraid of a mirror. Yeast infections lead to a chunkier-looking discharge.

But if you're on the phone with your doctor's office or at an appointment, don't self-diagnose. Instead of telling the nurse what you think you have, report your symptoms and how long they've been going on. That's way more helpful. You'll also want to share with your doctor any complicating circumstances: if you tried an over-the-counter remedy that didn't work, if you've got uncontrolled diabetes, if you have a compromised immune system, or if you tend to frequently get yeast infections. All these factors will influence what course of treatment your doctor chooses.

Protect yourself: Follow the 10 Vaginal Hygiene Commandments (see Principle #2) to avoid putting your Queen V at risk. You should also know other factors that can put you at risk, such as taking antibiotics, being overweight, or being pregnant, to name a few.

Treat yourself: If it's your first time getting a yeast infection or you get them only occasionally, I'll typically offer you an oral or intravaginal treatment like fluconazole (Diflucan) or butoconazole, respectively. For my patients who get recurrent yeast infections, I use a long-term therapy, which includes taking fluconazole once a week for eight weeks, then every other week for eight weeks, and then once a month for two to four months. I also recommend making probiotics a part of your vitamin routine to put good bacteria back in the vagina. I'll also suggest a ten- to twelve-day course of boric acid vaginal suppositories to reacidify the vagina.

Bacterial Vaginosis

What it is: First and foremost, it's not a sexually transmitted infection. BV occurs when the natural balance of bacteria in your vagina is thrown off. Suddenly there's too much of certain bacteria, resulting in a thin white, gray, or green discharge; a fishy vaginal smell; itching; and perhaps burning while urinating.

Sometimes confused with: Yeast infections (see above). Vaginitis, which is an umbrella term for several types of inflammation or infections that occur in the vagina, including yeast infections, BV, and trichomoniasis (see below).

How to tell the difference: The fishy odor and the type of discharge are usually dead giveaways, but some women have no signs when infected. That's problematic because even without symptoms, BV can cause problems like preterm delivery. It also may increase your chances of getting other infections such as STIs, post-surgery infections, or PID.

Protect yourself: Make sure you're taking a daily probiotic. Not having a healthy balance of bacteria in your vagina puts you at risk for BV. Don't douche, don't wash with scented soaps, and don't use scented tampons or pads. They could possibly upset the balance of bacteria in your vagina. Having a new sex partner or multiple sex partners can also increase your risk, so always use condoms.

Treat yourself: Sometimes your immune system will kick in and take care of BV all by itself. But given the complications it can cause, you're better off seeing your doctor to have it treated. If it's a one-off and this doesn't happen to you often, it can be treated with vaginal creams or pills. One of my favorite regimens includes clindamycin, metronidazole, and tinidazole. If you get recurrent BV, we'll use the same medications but for an extended period of time. I've also used boric acid suppositories to try to stop a resurgence.

Urinary Tract Infection

What it is: That feeling that you have to go all the time, you only pee a little bit when you do, and, ow, it burns. Most people think UTIs only involve the bladder, but they're actually more widespread than you realize. A UTI is an infection in any part of your system related to urination, such as your kidneys (which make urine), ureters (the muscular tubes that push urine from your kidneys to your bladder), your bladder (which holds urine until it is expelled), and your urethra (the short tube in your vagina that expels urine from your body).

Sometimes confused with: Yeast infections and sexually transmitted infections like chlamydia and herpes.

How to tell the difference: UTIs won't cause a discharge or result in herpes-like sores.

Protect yourself: Plenty of surprising behaviors can have you down for the count with a UTI, including having a lot of sex (honeymoon cystitis), using a diaphragm (it can hold bacteria inside your vagina, which is next door to the urethra), using unlubricated condoms (thanks to the friction), using spermicide, or simply having diabetes, sickle cell trait, or other chronic illnesses.

Try to avoid problems by urinating immediately before and after sex to expel any bacteria that may have gotten into your urethra. Drink plenty of water throughout the day to flush out your kidneys—however much you're drinking, up your intake. Try working cranberry supplements or unsweetened or low-sugar cranberry juice into your diet. The jury's still out on cranberry's effectiveness, but it may help thanks to an ingredient that prevents bacteria from sticking to the walls of your bladder. And, of course, don't forget to follow the 10 Vaginal Hygiene Commandments.

Not to scare you, but UTIs can be deadly, so don't ignore them. I've heard of pregnant patients with UTIs who disregarded the symptoms because they thought it was just part of carrying a child. The infection then traveled up to their kidneys and their lungs and they became septic and died. If you think you have a UTI, don't waste time drinking cranberry juice and hoping for the best. See a physician.

Treat yourself: If it's a one-off, call your doctor for treatment, which will likely include antibiotics and/or an office visit. If you frequently get UTIs, there may be an office visit, urine cultures, and extended antibiotic treatment. If you get frequent UTIs *associated with sex*, some doctors will prescribe antibiotic maintenance treatment, which will include one pill each day you have sex.

Chlamydia

What it is: This bacterial infection is spread through vaginal, anal, and oral sex by an infected partner—even if he's male and doesn't ejaculate. Despite the fact that more than a million cases of chlamydia are reported each year, nearly three million cases go undiagnosed and undetected. Why? A large number of people infected with chlamydia don't experience any symptoms.

Sometimes confused with: A UTI, yeast or vaginal infection, or gonorrhea. You might think that you've been working out too hard or lifting things that are too heavy. I've had a lot of women complain of horrible back pain only to find out a spreading chlamydia infection was the cause.

How to tell the difference: Get tested if you've had unprotected sex and several weeks later experience bleeding after sex or between periods; abnormal yellowish or foul-smelling vaginal discharge; pain or a burning sensation during sex or urination; nausea; and lower back or belly pain.

Infertility risk: Yes. Untreated, chlamydia can cause PID that can affect your ability to get pregnant.

Treat yourself: Often a silent STI, chlamydia can cause blindness in babies. That's one of the reasons why OB-GYNs routinely test pregnant patients for this STI—and others—to make sure they're not infected. It's very treatable with antibiotics once diagnosed by your doctor.

Gonorrhea

What it is: Before you ask, let me tell you right now: Yes, people are still getting gonorrhea. In fact, the number of cases reported in the United States in the past five years is on the rise with more than half a million people getting it in 2017. Gonorrhea, a bacterial infection, transmits when semen, pre-ejaculate, or vaginal fluids get on or inside your genitals, mouth, or anus. Researchers are still looking into whether you can get it just from kissing.

Sometimes confused with: UTI, vaginal infection, or chlamydia.

How to tell the difference: Possible symptoms include frequent urination with burning; an increase in vaginal bleeding or discharge; rectal itching, bleeding, or discharge; painful bowel movements; and even a fever. Symptoms can appear anywhere from two to fourteen days after having unprotected sex.

Infertility risk: Yes. Like chlamydia, it can lead to PID.

Treat yourself: Antibiotics from your doctor.

HIV/AIDS

What it is: Human immunodeficiency virus (HIV) attacks and damages your body's immune system. Over time, HIV can destroy so many cells that the body can't fight off infections and disease. Passed on through semen, vaginal fluids, anal mucus, blood, and breast milk, HIV can infect your body through cuts or sores in skin, mucous membranes (inside the vagina, rectum, and penis opening), as well as through shared needles or syringes. Unlike some other viruses, the human body can't get rid of HIV completely, but with certain medications, you can live a healthy life and lower or stop the chances of spreading the virus to others. Drugs developed to treat HIV can reduce the amount of the virus in your blood so much that it might not show up as detectable on tests, which means you can't transmit the virus through sex. If untreated, HIV can lead to acquired immunodeficiency syndrome (AIDS). People with AIDS have such badly damaged immune systems that they get an increasing number of serious opportunistic infections including tuberculosis, certain cancers, and brain disorders.

Sometimes confused with: The flu, a cold, sore throat, mononucleosis, or pneumonia.

How to tell the difference: You have to be tested. Symptoms also vary depending upon the disease's stage, but 40 to 90 percent of people with HIV experience flu-like symptoms within two to four weeks of infection. If HIV progresses to AIDS, you might experience rapid weight loss; extreme tiredness; recurring fever; prolonged swelling of lymph glands and reddish, brown, pink, or purplish blotches on or under the skin or inside the mouth, nose, or eyelids.

Infertility risk: Yes. Research has shown that HIV and drugs used to treat it can make it more difficult to get pregnant.

Treat yourself: Antiretroviral therapy (ART) isn't a cure, but it can stop the progression and reduce the amount of HIV in your body. The truth of the matter is that fear of HIV significantly decreased with the availability of better medications to manage it; it's no longer a death sentence. In fact, some treatments can get your viral load (the amount of HIV in your body) so low that it's almost undetectable. But you still need to use protection—no matter what type of sex you're engaging in—and talk to your partner about what they may be at risk for. I still see women in my practice who find out they're positive when they get pregnant. They're terrified for their babies. Don't presume by the way someone looks or how much money they make that they couldn't be positive. Know your own and your partner's status.

Hepatitis

What it is: Hepatitis means inflammation of the liver and is broken down into five types: A, B, C, D, and E. In terms of impact, all types of hepatitis affect the liver. In terms of transmission, there are key differences. Hep B is most likely to be spread through sex. While hep A and hep C can be sexually transmitted, the former is more commonly contracted through contaminated food and water. The latter is more often contracted from needles and syringes.

Sometimes confused with: Abdominal pain and gastrointestinal issues (diarrhea and vomiting), fatigue, or the flu.

How to tell the difference: Hepatitis A, B, or C may cause your skin and eyes to appear jaundiced and turn your urine a dark color.

Infertility risk: Yes. Research shows that hep B and C are linked to lower female fertility due to various causes such as tubal damage and premature decline in ovarian function.

Treat yourself: There are vaccines for hepatitis A and B that you likely got as a child to protect you from the infection. If you never got vaccinated or contracted another strain, your doctor will offer a vaccination.

Trichomoniasis

What it is: This infection is caused by a parasite that travels between partners during intercourse. It can be hard to tell if you're infected since only about 30 percent of those affected develop any symptoms. It's typically found to be more common in women than men, and trichomoniasis disproportionately affects African Americans.

Sometimes confused with: Genital inflammation, irritation, itching, or a UTI.

How to tell the difference: Trichomoniasis may come with a foul-smelling vaginal discharge that can be white, gray, yellow, or green. It's usually foamy, like the froth on a cup of gourmet coffee. When your doctor performs an internal exam, they may notice what we call a "strawberry cervix" because the infection changes its color and physical appearance. Pain with urination or during intercourse, vaginal redness, burning, and itching are also general signs.

Infertility risk: Possibly. In rare cases, it can cause PID.

Treat yourself: An antibiotic like metronidazole (Flagyl) or tinidazole (Tindamax).

Syphilis

What it is: A bacterial infection that enters the body through mucous membranes or torn or cut skin. Once inside the body, syphilis enters the bloodstream and attaches to cells, damaging organs over time. There are four stages in which untreated syphilis progresses: primary, secondary, latent, and tertiary (or late). The primary stage of syphilis is usually marked by the appearance of a single, painless, raised or elevated sore, known as a chancre, at the spot the bacteria entered your body. Although the sore will heal on its own anywhere between three and six weeks, syphilis can remain dormant in your body without detectable symptoms for many years. Untreated syphilis can cause major health problems and damage throughout your body.

Sometimes confused with: Warts, pimples, rashes, canker sores, or cold sores caused by oral herpes.

How to tell the difference: A syphilis sore is usually firm, round, and painless, though sometimes it can be open and wet. There's often only one sore.

Infertility risk: It doesn't appear syphilis poses a barrier to getting pregnant, but it can be passed on from mother to unborn baby. Congenital syphilis greatly increases risk of miscarriage, stillbirth, or newborn's death shortly after birth.

Treat yourself: While curable with antibiotics like penicillin, complications that may develop in later stages cannot be reversed with treatment.

Genital Herpes (See Principle #1)

One more thing: Back in Principle #1, I gave you a breakdown of the blisters and sores that can be caused by the herpes simplex virus. It's worth noting that not all outbreaks are visible. Your first sign may be flu-like symptoms, such as fever and chills.

Because many women have outbreaks around their period, be on the lookout for strange symptoms when it's that time of the month.

Genital Warts/HPV (See Principle #1)

One more thing: Back in Principle #1, I gave you the rundown on this extremely common sexually transmitted infection. With four out of five sexually active people being infected at some point in their lifetime, it's pretty ubiquitous. And there are forty different strains of the disease. Ready for the good news? Most infections go away on their own in a few years. Plus, there's a vaccine to protect you from nine of the most dangerous strains—the ones that stick around and are most often the cause of genital warts and cervical cancer. While the vaccination is *available* to people from nine to forty-five years old, it's only *recommended* by the Centers for Disease Control for girls ages eleven to twelve and women up to age twenty-six. The CDC recommends that women ages twenty-seven to forty-five who haven't been vaccinated make the decision with their doctor. I mention to my patients twenty-seven and up that the shots are an option but may not be covered by insurance. Once you've been exposed to a particular strain of HPV, the vaccine won't help you fight that strain—but can help prevent exposure to others. Plus, if you're a Virgin Mary or Sanctified Snatch who thinks you might not have been exposed at all and could still benefit, talk to your doctor about getting vaccinated.

WHAT'S LUBE GOT TO DO WITH IT?

Need a little help getting slippery when wet? There's more than one way to make sure your next sexual experience is smooth sailing. With the variety of sexual lubricants on the market today, you can find something that suits your Queen V to a T.

Silicone-based lubes are smooth, silky, hypoallergenic, waterproof, safe to use with latex condoms, and long lasting. The lubes shouldn't be used with silicone sex toys because the lube's silicone can ruin a silicone toy's surface, making it less sanitary.

Best for: Anal and vaginal sex with condoms, those with allergies or skin sensitivities, and shower or tub sex.

Water-based lubricants offer a non-greasy romp that won't badly stain your sheets. Since these lubes dry out faster, you may need to reapply during sex. Like silicone-based lubes, these are condom-compatible and won't break down the rubber. Though flavored water-based warming or cooling lubes might seem made for oral sex, certain flavors (think menthol or cinnamon) might cause your mouth to tingle, burn, or feel numb.

Best for: Anal or vaginal sex with condoms and sex toys.

Oil-based lubes provide slickness and contain fewer additives and preservatives. Any oil-based lubes or natural oils such as avocado, olive oil, or coconut should never be used with latex or polyisoprene condoms—they can cause a condom to degrade, slip, or break. And avoid lubes with petroleum and glycerin, which have been associated with higher rates of urinary and vaginal infections.

Best for: Partners who don't need to use condoms, oral sex, skin sensitivities, massage foreplay, and masturbation.

Hybrid lubes combine water and silicone formulas that provide slickness and don't absorb as quickly. They are also less sticky than a water-based lube. Hybrids sometimes taste bitter, so it may not be optimal for oral sex.

Best for: Longer lasting anal and vaginal sex, and shower or tub sex.

All-natural offerings are typically water-based and free of parabens, hormones, dyes, glycerin, alcohol, and fragrances. Many natural lubes boast aloe vera. If so, make sure it's 100 percent pure aloe vera since some aloe-infused products include ingredients or sugar that can cause vaginal irritation and yeast infections.

Best for: Vegans, people with sensitive skin or allergies, and oral sex.

WHAT'S YOUR QUEEN V'S FAVORITE CONDOM?

I want to change the conversation around wearing a condom. What if instead of thinking, "I have to use a condom," we all thought, "Wow, I get to use a condom!" What if we took the tension out of the moment of suiting up and instead infused it with the excitement of wrapping up a present for your V?

You could probably find a different type of condom for every type of sex you'd want to have, every person you'd want to have it with, and every day of the week! There are condoms for oral sex that are flavored like mint chocolate or tropical fruits. Condoms for your enhanced pleasure with ridges and bumps. Condoms that are "extra strong" for anal sex. Condoms that are fitted (for smaller guys who are surely gifted in other departments), and condoms that are bigger (for the well-endowed men who know how blessed they are).

One way to find the best condom for you is to treat them like candles or hand lotions and go to a store to inspect and sniff each one before deciding which to take home. But I suggest finding a brand you're interested in exploring and consider getting a variety pack of their condoms so you and your partner have a selection of different love gloves to test ride each night. In the meantime, here's the least you should know about the different materials they're made from:

- **Latex** is the most common material used for condoms and is capable of stretching a whopping 800 percent of its size. If you're worried about allergies to latex—or byproducts that may be in latex condoms—consider **polyurethane** or **polyisoprene**. These tend to be thinner, with users reporting they can feel more sensation using them. When used properly, all three will protect against pregnancy and sexually transmitted infections.

- **Lambskin** condoms are made from a sheep's intestines, so if you're focused on the environment, these biodegradable options may make you feel like you're doing Mother Nature a solid. Be aware that while they'll protect you from pregnancy, their more porous nature lets infections slip through. They *won't* protect you from STIs.

- If you're using a female condom, which conveniently puts you in control and can be inserted into your vagina up to eight hours before sex, it's likely made out of a rubbery material called **nitrile**. You have to be comfortable with your body to insert a female condom, so it's not something I see my Virgin Marys or Sanctified Snatches excited to do. It should also be noted that female condoms are a little more expensive than male condoms and may take a little getting used to.

Need some help putting one on? Go to Principle #6 for a visual guide.

TOUGH TALKS:
HOW TO TELL SOMEONE YOU HAVE AN STI

You already know that a new partner can bring out a different VP in you. You're not going to be the same person in bed with the college professor you met on Match as you would be with the starving artist you met on Tinder. There's something else that can bring out a different VP in you as well: leaving town.

I had a Mary Jane patient who uncovered the Notorious V.A.G. inside her when she went on vacation in the Caribbean. She was just visiting a guy friend but ended up bumping into another friend while taking a walk on the beach. Well, between the sun, sand, and sexy-sounding cocktails, she ended up in a threesome. A week later she was in my office complaining of discharge which ended up being a symptom of chlamydia. She had no idea who infected her or when it happened, but she owned it. Mary Jane felt horrible about putting her two friends at risk. What's more, she had to make not one but two phone calls to tell both of them they needed to get tested.

As soon as you find out that you have contracted a sexually transmitted infection, you must tell your partner(s). I know it's not easy and it requires putting on your big girl panties. But it's absolutely essential. Gather all the facts you know about the infection you've contracted, brace your partner(s) for a serious conversation, let them know what infection they may have gotten from you (or given you), and suggest they get tested.

If you're living with a long-term sexually transmitted infection like herpes or HIV, my advice is a little different. I've had patients tell me, "I met this guy and I wanted to be open and honest with him up-front, so I told him I had herpes. He never called me back." Honestly, I wouldn't either. You didn't allow your partner to get to know you as a person before finding out what was going on behind the scenes. If you meet someone and *immediately* start talking about your STIs, you're basically pushing them into someone else's arms. Instead, give the relationship time to grow so you know each other better. Then, before it escalates to sex, sit them down for a serious talk outside the bedroom. You can say something like, "I was diagnosed with herpes in college. I'm not having frequent outbreaks and I *do* know how to keep you safe." Honesty isn't the easiest, but it is always the best policy.

POINT OF V: STOP WITH THE SINS OF OMISSION

I love a woman who is in control of her emotions—and that's what protecting your Queen V is all about. What feels good for fifteen seconds can change the rest of your sexual life. I don't want you ladies making a permanent decision based on a temporary state of mind. So whether you're fingering, fisting, or something in between, be safe. Make sure you're not passing an infection on to someone else—and make sure your partner isn't passing an infection along to you. Ask them about their sexual health history and insist on using protection until you know it's safe not to. Sex is an incredibly beautiful thing, but you can't really enjoy what happens in bed until you get everything out on the table, so to speak. Let your relationship confessions be cathartic. Turn your struggle to speak up into strength of expression. And avoid any lies so you can focus on complete, passionate, and unconditional loving.

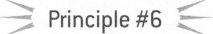

Principle #6

You Need a Platinum-Level Protection Plan—Even If You're Married

THE DELIVERY-DAY SURPRISE

I once had a Notorious V.A.G. patient with an unplanned pregnancy who spent nine months totally terrified of what was going to happen in the delivery room. Her fiancé was a light-skinned black man—but her side piece was an olive-skinned white guy. She had no idea which man had gotten her pregnant or what the baby was going to look like. And it haunted her until her delivery day when—you better praise Him—she pushed out a beautiful, smart baby that looked just like her soon-to-be husband. Or did it? She still wasn't 100 percent sure if it was his. To this day, I don't know if she ever found out.

I'm not trying to scare you with this story about the pitfalls of unplanned pregnancies. I am trying to give purpose to another woman's pain. If you got a chill reading about this woman because she sounds like you, know that you're not alone and your doctor might be able to help. There are ways to genetically test your baby in utero. Carefully consider that option with your doctor. (And if you do move forward, test your lover's DNA, *not* your primary partner's—just in case.)

If this baby daddy drama doesn't sound like you now, let's make sure it *never* sounds like you in the future. Taking chances with pregnancy and sexually transmitted infections is literally like playing a game of Russian roulette. As the "game" progresses, your chances of something going terribly wrong increase. Let my Notorious V.A.G.'s story be a cautionary tale that moves you to action by getting a platinum-level protection plan

against accidental pregnancy and STIs. And, no, I'm not just talking to
the single women out there. I believe every woman—married or solo—
should have a plan in place for her Queen V, and the first step is deciding which contraceptive (or which contraceptives) is best for you. (For my
trans readers, you might want to skip ahead a few pages to where we talk
about condoms for a refresher on the dos and don'ts of use.)

PICKING THE BEST BIRTH CONTROL FOR YOU

When it comes to choosing who'll be in the "royal guard" protecting your
Queen V from sperm, there are no right or wrong choices. There are, however, six divisions of protection:

- Barrier methods (cervical caps, condoms, and more)
- Hormonal options (these include the pill as well as the patch,
  the ring, and more)
- Natural planning (like fertility awareness methods, or FAMs)
- IUDs (hormonal and nonhormonal)
- Emergency contraception
- Sterilization

Virgin Marys can rest assured because abstinence is the only
100 percent effective form of birth control, and—assuming you're not
even rubbing up against anyone—it'll keep your Queen V free of sexually transmitted infections as well. For everyone else intent on hitting the
sheets, you'll need to pick one of the methods below:

Breastfeeding

Lactational amenorrhea (no period due to breastfeeding) magically kicks
in when you nurse your baby exclusively every four hours during the day
and every six hours at night. The practice stops you from ovulating, so it's
98 percent effective. You can see from these numbers, you've got to be on

top of nursing like you're punching a clock at a job you desperately need. Unlike any other contraceptive, it's only an option for a short period of time: the first six months of your baby's life.

Planned Parenthood lists this as a valid form of birth control, but I personally don't advocate for it. Maybe that's because I only see patients when they've made a mistake with it and ended up pregnant. I had a Virgin Mary who came to see me because she was having trouble producing milk for her new baby. Turned out her levels were low because she'd gotten pregnant again. She'd fallen off schedule with breastfeeding and had to start planning for baby number two sooner than she expected.

Cervical Cap

Ready to get up close and personal with your cervix? When inserted (by you) into your vagina, this barrier method covers your cervix so sperm can't enter your uterus. It must be used with spermicide (see description below) and left in place for at least six hours after sex. It's smaller than a diaphragm and you can keep the cap in for forty-eight hours. If you have sex multiple times during that period, be sure to insert more spermicide into your vagina. Cervical caps require a prescription since they're not one-size-fits-all. Cap effectiveness is 71 percent for women who've had a baby and 86 percent for women who've never given birth.

Internal Condom (FC2)

Commonly known as the female condom, this *single-use*, soft plastic pouch comes lubricated and goes inside your Queen V—but many people have been using it for safe anal sex as well. The good news: it puts you in control of protection. I had a very sweet Sanctified Snatch who got romantically involved with a man from her church while she and her husband were doing a trial separation. The one time she had sex with her new guy, he pulled out a condom and acted like he was putting it on. But the next day she found an unwrapped condom lying in her bed. He swore to her that he used protection but she knew it wasn't true when she tested positive for an STI . . . that she eventually passed on to her husband when they rec-onciled. The moral of the story is that you should reach, rub, and check to see that the condom is on your partner—or use an internal condom yourself.

Now, you have to be comfortable enough with your body to insert it. It goes in like a tampon with the condom's inner ring fitting around your cervix while the external ring remains outside for your partner's penis to enter. Doubling up won't give you any extra protection, so don't try to use a male condom with it. The female condom is made of nitrile, a latex alternative, and it's about 79 percent effective.

External Condom

Commonly known as the male condom, these cover your partner's penis during sex. Don't just let your man tear it open and go. Check the wrapper for any damage, check the condom for any discoloration, and always keep an eye on your man (with a smile) to make sure he's putting it on properly. Since condoms can tear, break, or slip off—hence all the attention you're paying when it's put on—they're 85 percent effective and can only be used once.

I've had several Coochie-Chondriacs tell me that condoms aren't an option because "he won't use them." I think to myself, "Excuse me?" Don't ask. You have to insist. Don't give your partner the power to put you at risk for pregnancy or STIs. I understand that women might not want their man to think they're implying he has an infection or they don't trust him, so you can be playful about it, but you have to be adamant too. "No condom, no cookie, honey." Have a little fun by helping him put it on while you're at it.

Diaphragm

Just like the cervical cap, a diaphragm is a soft cup that acts as a roadblock to sperm trying to travel to your cervix and uterus. It also needs to be used with spermicide and requires a prescription. It's larger than a cervical cap and about 88 percent effective.

Fertility Awareness Methods

FAMs, also called natural family planning or the rhythm method, refer to ways to track your menstrual cycle so you can recognize when you're ovulating and most likely to conceive. (Yes, there's an app for that. You could just break out a pen and a piece of paper too.) There are several methods such as taking your temperature each morning—basal body temperature rises during ovulation—and checking the color and texture of your cervical mucus so you can either abstain from sex or use another method of birth control on fertile days. FAMs are 76 to 88 percent effective and work better when multiple methods are used together.

Implant (Nexplanon)

The biggest question that I get about this tiny, matchstick-size, long-acting, reversible contraceptive (LARC) is: "Is it going to hurt?" The answer is no. I give patients a numbing shot before inserting the implant into the upper part of their nondominant arm. It takes a minute or two. You might feel sore at the site for a couple of days, but that should go away. With a 99 percent effective rate, the birth control implant offers one of the safest, longest-lasting, mistake-proof choices. It works by releasing the hormone progestin into your body. Progestin interrupts ovulation and also thickens cervical mucus so it's harder for sperm to reach an egg if you were to still ovulate.

The side effects are different for everyone: some women report having shorter periods or no bleeding at all, while others experience irregular bleeding, weight gain, or possibly acne. It can last for up to three years, so after you get it, you can forget it. Want to get pregnant? No problem, your doctor can take it out at any time and you can start trying right away.

Intrauterine Device (IUD)

For your consideration, meet the second most popular form of contraception I prescribe or insert in my office. It's another LARC. This small, Y- or T-shaped device with string hanging from the bottom protects you from getting pregnant for three to ten years and provides a more than 99 percent effective rate. (By the way, if Big Daddy can feel the string while you're having sex and it bothers him, go back to your provider and have them trim it.)

IUDs come in two types: nonhormonal copper and hormonal ones made with levonorgestrel (progestin). It is thought that the copper produces an inflammatory reaction that's toxic to sperm, making it almost impossible to reach an egg. Nonhormonal copper IUDs can be very effective as emergency contraception when placed within five days of unprotected sex (but they're rarely inserted for this specific purpose). Hormonal IUDs thicken cervical mucus to stop sperm from entering the uterus, thin the lining of the uterus, and can stop ovulation.

It's worth noting that IUDs need to be inserted and removed by a physician. I've had a few Coochie-Chondriacs come in after attempting to remove it themselves because they just couldn't get comfortable with something being put inside them. Unfortunately, that's a bad idea, particularly if there are any complications preventing an easy removal. You could potentially leave a piece of the IUD stuck in your uterus or cervix. Let your doctor handle it, ladies.

The Patch

The hormones estrogen and progestin enter the skin through a plastic square adhesive (which looks like a big Band-Aid) to stop ovulation and thicken cervical mucus so sperm can't fertilize an egg. You can wear a patch on your stomach, butt, back, or outer upper arm every week for three weeks, and on your patch-free week, you should get your period. Put a new patch on to start the four-week cycle again even if you're still bleeding. I tell patients to check and make sure their patch is there every day—and to be mindful of it when you're applying lotion or oil to your body, or swimming or getting sweaty while exercising. You'll need a prescription from your doctor for the patch, and it's about 91 percent effective.

Pill

Even though there are much easier options, everybody loves the pill. Four out of five sexually active women have used the pill at some point in their lives. It's the most popular contraceptive in my practice. The birth control pill stops fertilization by halting ovulation so there's no egg for a sperm to find. There are two types: combination (estrogen and progestin) or progestin-only pills that typically come in a 21- or 28-day pack. Birth control pills have a 91 to 99 percent effectiveness rate. Missing pills or getting off schedule can result in an increased risk of getting pregnant, so if that happens, use a backup form of protection. Every woman is different, so some experience side effects (like weight gain, acne, or irregular bleeding) and others don't.

Ring (NuvaRing)

Just like all the other contraceptives you insert yourself, the ring requires you to be comfortable with your vagina. I don't think a lot of Virgin Marys, Sanctified Snatches, or Coochie-Chondriacs reading this will be interested in the monthly self-insertion and removal this small, flexible ring you wear inside your vagina requires. It releases pregnancy-preventing hormones absorbed by the vaginal lining to halt ovulation. You wear the ring for three weeks, remove it, and after seven ring-free days, put in a new one. The ring is 91 percent effective. If you find you're still spotting while using it, you can still use tampons. Just be careful you don't dislodge the ring when you take out the tampon.

Speaking of dislodging, it's not common, but I have heard of it happening.

One of my patients found her ring in the bed when she was changing her sheets. Ordinarily you can just rinse off the ring with lukewarm water and reinsert it. But this woman hadn't made her bed in several days, and by the time she came into my office she was pregnant. (Yup! Pregnant!) This isn't a slam against the ring—which is incredibly convenient. It's actually a nudge to make your bed (or check your vagina) regularly if you get one.

Shot/Injection (Depo-Provera)

At one point in 2010, a whopping 23 percent of women had tried using this form of birth control. My patients either love it or hate it. They love it because of the convenience. One poke of a progestin injection and you're done. They hate it because of side effects like weight gain or irregular bleeding—which we can try to address with a supplemental hormonal method like the patch, ring, or estrogen pill.

The injection is typically given in the privacy of your doctor's office every three months and suppresses ovulation and thickens cervical mucus. It's 94 percent effective if you remember to get a shot on time (anywhere between ten and fifteen weeks since your last one), but the longer you go past the recommended twelve weeks between shots, the greater your chance of getting pregnant. If you prefer to give yourself the shot at home, ask your provider if that's an option. Some will allow you to have a family member administer the shot if, for example, the person is a nurse. I don't recommend this method for women who want to get pregnant soon as it can take up to eighteen months for the hormones to clear out of your body.

Spermicide

Spermicides are chemicals you put into your vagina that kill sperm or stop it from traveling. You can buy spermicide in many forms, such as cream, gel, film, foam, and suppositories over the counter at drugstores. By itself, spermicide is only 71 percent effective, so it's best if you use it each time you have sex and combine it with another method, such as a condom.

Sponge (Today Sponge)

Here's one patients are usually mentioning to *me*—not the other way around. Think of this soft, squishy, spermicide-infused piece of foam like a cervical cap or diaphragm. It works the same way but it is shaped a little differently, available over the counter, and disposable. For women who've never given birth, sponges are about 88 percent effective. If you've had a child, the sponge is about 76 percent effective. You need to leave the sponge in place for at least six hours after sex and it's only good for one twenty-four-hour period once it's inside your vagina.

Tubal Ligation

While 72 percent of women who use contraceptives choose nonpermanent methods, that leaves about a quarter of you (28 percent) who don't. The majority of those women opt for this surgical procedure, also known as female sterilization or "getting your tubes tied." It is closing or blocking your fallopian tubes. After getting your tubes tied, you can still get your period but you can't conceive. The procedure can be reversed, but your chances of getting pregnant depend upon whether your doctor used clips or rings to block segments of your tubes rather than cauterization. It's one of the most effective (99 percent) and commonly used methods of contraception, especially in women ages forty to forty-nine.

Withdrawal

Withdrawal happens when a man pulls out before he ejaculates. Sperm can be released before the man exits the vagina, so it's only effective 78 percent of the time, and that's if no semen or pre-ejaculate gets near the vagina or vulva at all. It's often recommended that you use another form of birth control along with the withdrawal method in case of a slipup or leakage of sperm during sex.

DECISIONS, DECISIONS

Three things you and your doctor should take into consideration before picking a method of protection:

Your medical history. If you have an autoimmune disease (like lupus), I'd steer you away from a hormonal birth control method that could negatively impact your chronic illness. Women who are prone to deep vein thrombosis (DVT), for example, shouldn't be on a combination (estrogen and progestin) birth control pill, which could increase their chances of a pulmonary embolism.

Your lifestyle habits. Can't remember to call your mom every day? Chances are remembering to take a birth control pill every day won't work out for you either. But an IUD you don't have to think about for up to ten years could. Haven't quit smoking yet? A combination hormonal contraceptive like the patch isn't for you. But a progestin-only pill, nonhormonal IUD, or barrier method could be a good choice.

Your age. All estrogen-based methods are more of a concern for women thirty-five and older due to the increased risk of DVTs.

7 REASONS TO USE HORMONAL BIRTH CONTROL (THAT ACTUALLY HAVE NOTHING TO DO WITH PREGNANCY)

One of my Notorious V.A.G. patients came in a few years back worried about a terrible-smelling green discharge. After testing her, I found out that she had trichomoniasis . . . and that she was pregnant. And here's the catch: this Notorious V.A.G. was in a committed relationship with her lesbian partner. She'd never had sex with a man before. But she'd had a crazy little one-night-stand with a man she met in a bar, and boom! That's right, ladies. First time out and batting 1000. There's a happy ending to this story: she and her partner decided to keep and raise the blessing of a baby together. But the movie doesn't always end that way. Now, I'm not suggesting that lesbians use hormonal birth control just in case they have a wild night. But there are plenty of other reasons to get a prescription even if you're not strictly-dickly.

1. **You're just plain tired of surfing the crimson tide.** There's no medical reason that you need to have a period, so you can certainly go ahead and use continuous hormonal contraception to stop it.
2. **Your acne is out of control.** Certain brands of combination birth control pills are also approved by the Food and Drug Administration for dealing with breakouts.
3. **You haven't got time for the pain.** Who wouldn't want to say goodbye to being doubled over with an aching uterus every month?
4. **You're sold on the health benefits.** Oral contraceptives have been shown to reduce your risk of certain forms of cancer— including endometrial and ovarian. (Unfortunately, they increase your risk of breast and cervical cancer.) They can also reduce anemia, infections of the reproductive system, and good old bad-mood premenstrual syndrome (PMS).
5. **You're tired of head games.** For women who experience menstrual migraines, using continuous birth control can level out the hormonal fluctuations that spark these headaches.
6. **You're going through perimenopause.** Some women find that taking low-dose birth control pills during the years when their ovaries start to shut down can help with hot flashes, mood swings, and more.
7. **You don't identify as female.** If getting periods every month is a dreaded reminder of the gender you were assigned at birth, there are plenty of continuous contraceptive options without estrogen that can stop menstruation. If you feel awkward just having to sit in a gynecologist's office, talk to your doctor about LARCs.

HOW TO PUT ON A CONDOM

Slipping on a "raincoat" is not like riding a bicycle. If you've been out of the game for a while, you actually can forget—and so can your man. So while it might be tempting to lie back and let him suit up solo, remember your Queen V is depending on you. Before your date night, brush up on your love glove technique by practicing with a dildo, a banana, or a cucumber.

The first thing you want to do is check the packaging. Make sure it isn't past its expiration date and that the wrapper doesn't look damaged in any way. If it's been floating around at the bottom of your purse for months, it's probably not in good shape. If everything looks good, carefully open the package. Don't use anything that could tear the condom

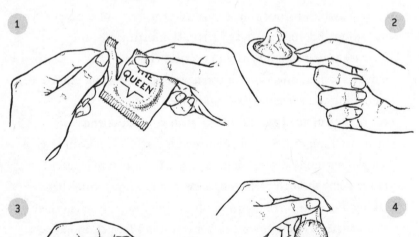

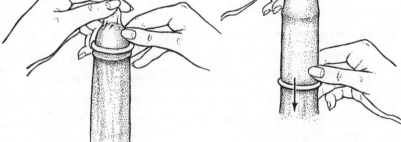

itself, like your teeth (sexy, but sharp), super-sharp nails (love those rhinestones, but c'mon), or scissors (pretty self-explanatory here).

Next, here's where the technique comes in. Grab the tip between your thumb and your forefinger—that leaves space for semen to collect and eliminates a bubble—and then place it on the head of your man's erect penis. Unroll the condom all the way to the base of your partner's penis. If it's hard to unroll, you might have it inside out.

After you get your ooh-ooh-ooh on, you want to avoid spilling what's inside the condom or losing it inside you. Once your partner ejaculates—but before his penis gets soft—make sure he holds the rim while pulling out of you and then turns away from you while removing the condom. Make sure the condom is intact by inspecting it from tip to base. Look for any missing pieces, tears, or holes.

SOS! YOU LOST THE CONDOM—OR IT BROKE

1. **Ask for help.** It actually might be easier for your partner to reach inside you to fish out what got left behind. Of course, you can try as well but he's got some angle advantages on you. If there's any question as to whether you've gotten the whole thing out, make an appointment with your doctor. Your fingers can't always reach as far as I can. I can do a speculum exam (you know, those cold "spoons" to take a look inside your vagina) to either reassure you there's nothing left inside or remove what was left.

2. **Consider EC.** If you're worried about pregnancy, emergency contraceptives (EC) can help. It's important to note that EC are not for abortions. They stop a pregnancy before it starts. Within five days of unprotected sex, you can take a one-dose pill (like Ella—which requires a prescription—or Plan B, Next Choice, and others that are available over the counter) or you could have your doctor place a copper-T IUD inside you. I recommend one-dose pills because getting a copper IUD is very expensive

and a procedure you need to make an appointment for. It's a smaller window and less effective, but within three days of unprotected sex or a condom mishap, you can also take more than one birth control pill to prevent pregnancy. You'll have to talk to your doctor about how many pills of your particular brand to take and how many doses you'll need. Effectiveness varies according to the method and when you take it, but could be up to 99 percent—that's for the IUD in particular.

3. **Talk about testing.** If you're even thinking about the possibility you got an STI, come up with a plan for testing with your doctor to see where you stand.

4 THINGS YOU SHOULD NEVER DO WITH A CONDOM

1. **Don't use it more than once.** Just like losing your virginity, it's one and done.

2. **Don't take it off in the middle of the action.** For some reason, a lot of you aren't suiting up for the whole game. One study found that about 25 percent of women who had used a condom in the past month said it was only on their partner "part of the time" during intercourse. Part-time coverage won't give you full-time protection. Your man has to slip on that love glove when his penis gets erect and not take it off until he pulls out of you.

3. **Don't use flavored condoms for intercourse.** Come on, now. You know those are just for oral sex and your Queen V won't be happy with flavored or scented shenanigans that could lead to a yeast infection.

4. **Don't assume the one you bought will fit.** In this case, size *does* matter. Which is why condoms come in a variety of lengths, widths, and shapes—some leaving extra room at the head. There are companies that will custom-size them for you. So shop around.

WHY YOUR QUEEN V NEEDS A PROTECTION PLAN

Getting tested for a sexually transmitted infection can be just as anxiety-inducing at forty-six as it is at sixteen. You may be trying to play it cool, but inside your mind is frantically racing: Am I sure he used a condom? Was that a pimple on her or something else? That drama isn't just for the teenagers who come into my office because they "forgot" to use a condom. Or all the single ladies who had one-night-stand "whoops!" moments. It stirs up in wives who have a little butterfly in their mind that something just ain't quite right at home with the hubs too. Yes, at least once a week, a married woman will sit down in my office and tell me she wants to get tested for STIs.

Sometimes the wives are just saying yes to the routine testing that comes with their annual visit. Other times, they're requesting it because mistakes were made. Maybe they saw a sexy text message on their partner's phone from a number they didn't recognize. Or found an expensive gift that wasn't meant for them. Or got a tip from an eagle-eyed friend who believes that if you see something, you better say something. No matter how it happens, thankfully they come to me to get checked out. (If your mind is telling you "yes," "maybe," or "why not?" then just do it. Get tested.)

I'm "old school" and I've always believed that marriage is a monogamous relationship. But I also know there is a new way of doing math. You can never trust someone 100 percent of the time. About 75 percent of the time, the person who doesn't deserve trust is my patient's partner—but about 25 percent of the time it's my patient. I get Notorious V.A.G.s, Mary Janes, and Coochie-Chondriacs who have stepped out on their significant others more than I'd like to admit. And that stepping out can lead to more than just STIs. It can also bring a baby into the world. So it pays to have a comprehensive protection plan.

Think about it: when you buy an expensive new cell phone, a sixty-inch television, or (seriously) a pair of headphones, the store clerk usually tries to upsell you and asks if you want to buy a protection plan in case it breaks or gets stolen. But when was the last time you thought about a protection plan for your Queen V? Unlike a laptop, she's harder to fix and impossible to replace. She'll be around a lot longer than your kitchen appliances, and she's a lot more important when it comes to dining in (or, heh, eating out). Plus, your Queen V protection plan is usually pretty cheap, if not completely free thanks to health insurance. You'll never be able to control someone else's actions in this world, but you can control your own. Get the best protection for your Queen V based on your relationship status by following one of the checklists below.

The "24/7" Support Protection Plan

- You're a happily married woman
- You're unmarried and in a committed relationship

√ Pick a Birth Control Method (Or Two) with Your Partner

Until you're ready to start making some beautiful babies, you and your partner need to talk about pregnancy prevention. The only methods that prevent both STIs and pregnancy are the male and female condom. But most couples I know kick barrier methods to the curb once they commit to each other. There are tons of other options with different efficacy rates (see the list above). If you're in a long-term relationship, one of the most important considerations will be how soon you want to have children—or if you want to have kids at all.

√ The Moment You Suspect, Get Checked

If at any point in your relationship you're worried about your partner stepping out on you, get tested. If you notice your partner's penis or vagina doesn't look, smell, or feel the same, get tested. Don't wait. Remember, you don't have to have sex to get an STI. Your partner could have a moment of weakness and just kiss someone, or they could feel innocent because they received oral sex but never returned the favor. Your man could've been hot-dogging someone (that's when you rub your penis between another person's butt cheeks) but never penetrated them. All these acts can transmit STIs to your partner. And your partner can bring those STIs home to you.

If you never got tested before having unprotected sex with your partner, it's still worthwhile to do so now. As you know from Principle #5, it's not uncommon to have an STI that doesn't show any signs. Your partner could be infected, not know it, and pass that infection on to you. But more important, this test serves as a baseline. It shows that you were STI-free at one point in time, should something change in the future.

The "Accident Forgiveness" Protection Plan

- You're single with a new partner
- You're single with a partner who has been unfaithful
- You're married and your partner has been unfaithful

√ Get Tested. Like, Yesterday.

You might be confused about why I'm lumping new partners in with unfaithful partners. It's not a judgment. It's just that your protection plans happen to be the same. Every woman in this category isn't clear on her partner's STI status. If you're starting a relationship, go to your doctor, tell them you've just met someone new, and request STI testing. If you know you have an STI (like herpes), there's no need for a retest unless you are planning to share and discuss this information. (By the way, this is the best icebreaker for that topic.) But exams like this are good to have on record in case you have a situation where the condom breaks or there's some spillage in the future. When you get your results, share them with your partner and ask to see theirs in return.

√ Put Your Faith in Paper

Don't have unprotected intercourse until you see your partner's test results. Get proof. Like I told you, some STIs don't show signs. It may not be that your partner is trying to trick you or is too embarrassed to speak up. They may not know what they have.

Timing is important. You shouldn't be having that conversation once you get into bed. Before you feel like you're entering into the zone when sex will be part of the relationship, there should be a talk about protection from STIs and pregnancy. Say "Because I care enough about you to protect you against STIs I may not be aware of—and I know you'd want the same—we should get tested." Make it about both of you.

If your partner has been unfaithful, you don't have to dress this conversation up and make it look pretty. Just insist on testing. Infidelity took away your options and now it's going to take away theirs. When your partner cheats, it's all the more important that you look out for your Queen V—because they sure didn't.

√ Get Comfortable Shutting Down Condomless Sex

Just like anyone holding court with a queen for the first time—or after a huge mistake—your partner is going to have to suit up and be on his best behavior. Just tell them: "No glove? No love. No paper? No nookie without protection." Don't cave and don't give in. Even if you think you're too tired at the end of the night to insist. Even if you've been out partying together and you don't want to ruin the moment. Even if you're about to have incredible makeup sex and you don't want to pour water on these red-hot flames. Until you know the results of those tests, do not put your Queen V at risk.

√ Always Have Condoms and/or Dental Dams on Hand

God bless the woman who has her own. She'll never have to miss out on sex because her partner didn't come packing (I mean condoms!).

√ Pick a Birth Control Method That Has Your Back

If you're using condoms, think about a backup method (in case the condom breaks) and what you'll want to be on next (if and when you quit condoms). See the list above for a variety of different options. You might think about alternatives that protect you from STIs (like switching from the male to the female condom so you're in control) or how often you'll have to manage your birth control (daily, weekly, monthly, etc.).

The "Complete Coverage" Protection Plan

- You're in a relationship and you've been unfaithful
- You're married and you've been unfaithful
- You have multiple current partners
- You're in an open relationship

√ Get Tested—At the Right Time

Had a momentary—or all-night—lapse of judgment? Whether you fess up or fake the world's worst migraine or yeast infection for the next few weeks, you must put off having unprotected sex with your partner until you're in the clear. (I'll leave it to you to figure out how to handle that situation. But it's not fair to put them at risk.) In the meantime, call your doctor and schedule an appointment to get tested ASAP.

If you and your partner are in an open relationship and not using protection—or if you've decided to have multiple current partners—you'll want to get tested every three to four months. You also need to accept that you're skydiving with a parachute you refuse to open. Someone might come along, grab you, and open theirs. Or you both could free fall to the ground.

√ Develop a Strategy

One of my Notorious V.A.G.s described her sex life as if she were the general manager of a basketball team. There was a captain of the team—that was her main squeeze. But there were two power forwards, a shooting guard, and a center who also showed her a good time. "Everybody except the captain of the team has to use a condom," she told me confidently. But

I still recommended testing for her at least twice a year (sometimes more) because condoms don't keep you safe from infections that can be transmitted by kissing someone. And no matter how skilled a general manager you think you are, no one uses condoms properly 100 percent of the time. I'm not saying this is the right strategy for everyone, but if you're going to be playing (or managing) the field, you definitely need to develop a playbook of your own—and tell your doctor about it.

√ Take a Pregnancy Test As Soon As You Miss a Period

There's only so much I can do to help you avoid who's-the-daddy drama if you're juggling multiple relationships without protection. Once you think (just think) you could be pregnant, shut down any uncertainty by taking a test. As soon as you confirm you are pregnant, it's crunch time. See your OB-GYN as soon as possible to determine who the father of your child is. You can do noninvasive testing after your eighth week of pregnancy.

After three different paternity tests came up negative, one of my Notorious V.A.G.s basically gave up on figuring out the identity of her kid. "Who else could it be?" I asked her. "I have no idea," she replied. "I was so sure it was one of those three." If you're out here like that, taking a pregnancy test sooner rather than later can help you keep track of your partners and have a firm answer for your kid down the road.

POINT OF V: RECLAIM YOUR POWER

Every so often, a patient will look at me stunned and say, "What do you mean 'pregnant'?" They've missed the signs, they didn't think it could happen to them, they were careless about contraceptives, and they're genuinely surprised. If you upgrade your Queen V to a platinum protection plan, your chances of getting caught off guard will drop faster than your undies on Valentine's Day. You won't have to worry about pregnancy because you'll be on the best birth control for your Queen V. You won't have to stress about STIs because you'll know how to advocate for getting tested and avoid transmission. Let my advice in this chapter help you to protect your Queen V—without offending your partner. (Bonus: you're also saving your partner from potentially unwanted parenthood or an infection you might not know you have.) Most of all, let this chapter empower you to take back control of your body—without being totally controlling. But then again, power can be pretty sexy.

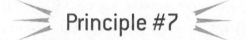

Principle #7

Always Plan Your Trip to His Netherlands

NOT EVERY PICTURE IS WORTH A THOUSAND WORDS

For the last twenty-something years, the only grown man's penis I've been up close and personal with is my husband Curtis's. I spend about 95 percent of my time catering to Queen Vs—not scrutinizing King Ps—unless we're talking about the baby boys I circumcise after delivery. That's why I was slightly out of my element when a prim and proper patient came into my office and pulled out her phone to show me a photo of her boyfriend's penis. Yes, you read that right. This woman scrolled past images of her adorable nieces, group photos with her church friends, and shots of fancy dinners to tap and zoom in on a picture of her man's frank and beans.

"Do you see that, Dr. Jackie?" she asked nervously, pointing to a darkened ring around his shaft with a tiny bump on it. "What do you think that is?"

Some pictures are worth a thousand words, but this one was only worth one: "Nothing," I told her after giving it as close a look as I could. The ring was likely a scar left from circumcision and the bump didn't have any of the distinct coloring or odd shape that would give me a reason to be concerned. I calmed her fears by saying that, judging from the picture, she didn't need to worry. But I also let her know that if she wanted to be 100 percent sure, she should tell her man to see his own doctor. Like I said, I don't see a lot of adult magic sticks.

Now, if you're like me, you probably have the same question on your mind right now that I did back in that exam room: How in *the world* did this woman get this penis pic on her phone in the first place? Was my patient a buttoned-up, Burberry-wearing Sanctified Snatch by day and a sexting-loving, satin-sheets-sleeping Notorious V.A.G. by night? Did she lift the covers and snap a photo of her man's third leg while he was sleeping? Had she demanded to know what was going on with his wedding tackle before it got tangled up in her bush, so they took the picture together? We may never know.

At the end of the day, it didn't really matter. My wish for you all is that you're confident enough to request testing (for yourself and from your partner) before having unprotected intercourse. But I know that not every woman feels empowered to ask that of her partner. Or to speak up when she sees something doesn't look right on him. I also know that even if you're using a condom or just having outercourse, it's still possible to get a sexually transmitted infection. So I have to say I was pleased that this Sanctified Snatch was using all her resources to look out for her health and protect her Queen V.

If you're not bold enough to question the safety of his swing set, you can still get answers for yourself. Your meekness does not have to be your weakness. I'm not suggesting that everyone start taking penis pics on the sly, but I do have some techniques for helping you figure out if your man's P-train needs to be taken out of service for a little while.

I know that not every woman reading this book is interested in having sex with a man. I'm also aware that my transsexual readers will already be familiar with a lot of this content. But since we've covered what to look for on vaginas, it's important to address what to look for on penises too. It's good info for *everyone*: Remember that lesbian patient of mine who ended up pregnant from a one-night stand with a guy she met at a bar? So let's start at the very beginning by talking about what the penis looks like in the first place.

MEETING A KING P

Some of my Virgin Marys, Sanctified Snatches, and Mary Janes are just starting to get comfortable looking at their own Queen Vs. Now here I come, pushing you even further, by asking you to lock eyes with some one-eyed monsters too. I know that might be a big ask. But I wouldn't ask if it wasn't important—as my Coochie-Chondriacs and my Notorious V.A.G.s already know. There's no shame in upping your sex education game. There's only power in it. Penises come in all different sizes and textures, and they can vary in color depending on genetics, surgery (if you're with a trans man), and more. But some things will usually be the same. Here's a quick anatomy lesson on your man's third leg.

> **Glans.** This is the tip or the head of his penis and it's a lot like your clitoris in that it's the most sensitive part of his member. Unlike your clitoris, three things (pre-ejaculate, semen, and urine) come out of the glans through a hole at its center connected to a thin tube called the urethra.
>
> **Foreskin.** If your man isn't circumcised, he'll have this patch of skin that covers the head of his penis. When his member gets erect, it will retract and expose the glans. When he's flaccid, it will cover the glans. But—heads up, ladies—he has to pull back the foreskin to clean his penis properly or else bacteria, dead skin cells, and oil can build up to cause an odor or inflammation.
>
> If your man is circumcised, that means that his foreskin has been surgically removed. The procedure is usually done for religious, cultural, or hygienic reasons. When performed on a newborn, the surgery is usually quick and simple. When the decision is made later in life, it's a bit more complicated and can take longer for guys to heal.
>
> Circumcision rates are down in the US, with about 58 percent of boys going under the knife, according to the last report, from

2010. That means your chances of seeing some foreskin are on the rise and there's nothing to be freaked out about. When my patients do complain to me, I remind them that some women tell me the sex is better. Kind of like he's ribbed for your pleasure.

Frenulum: It's where the foreskin meets the underside of the penis. Even if your man has been circumcised, he may still have all or part of his frenulum intact. (Pro tip: use the frenulum as an excuse to check your man out. Tell him you're curious to see how much he has left after circumcision.) Along with the glans, some guys say it's a highly sensitive part of the penis (yet another justification for some eyes-wide-open exploring).

Shaft: It's the entire length of your man's penis from where it meets his gut all the way to his glans. When a guy gets an erection, vessels that run through his shaft fill with blood, causing his penis to go from relaxed to a rocket ready for take-off.

Scrotum: Just a medical term for balls . . . or bro-varies . . . or the family jewels. These sensitive bags of skin hold your man's testicles, which is where sperm and hormones are produced.

YOU STARTED WITH THE MIRROR ON THE FLOOR, BUT NOW . . .

It's time to talk about the rod in the room. Back in Principle #1, I laid out all the reasons that you should grab a mirror and give your Queen V a once-over. Now I'm asking you to take a long, hard (wink wink) look at your man's naked King P. (Don't worry, I'll explain how to get a look later.) The reasons for taking a peek at his King P are pretty much the same as the ones I shared for looking at your Queen V.

But while you can silently stare at your own vagina, silently staring at your guy's penis will make him feel like he's naked in front of a crowd of laughing teenage girls. More than likely, no man's going to stand, sit, or lie there for that. So I'm helping you get the conversation going. For every empowering reason that I want you checking him out, I've given you the exact words you'll want to use while you're getting your looks in. (You're welcome.)

Empowering Reason: Prevention

What to Say: "Oh, honey. Hold on a second. What's that?"

If you two haven't gotten tested for sexually transmitted infections, this is your chance to look for signs of one. And if you see something, you definitely need to say something. Don't just think to yourself, "I'll do it next time." Next time will be too late. Hey, a few minutes later could be too late. You're helping your man out too. Some guys honestly have no idea they've got a problem between their legs. The sooner you tell him, the better off he'll be. Some sexually transmitted infections are more easily treated when they're caught early.

I don't want to tell you to lie, but if you truly can't bring yourself to ask "What's this?" or admit "I don't know about that bump," then I'll say it's time to get creative. Find a reason not to go down yonder, like saying you just started your period or things are moving too fast for you. Whatever defense you choose, don't just downgrade your sexual activity of choice. Stop all action together. "Outercourse" can be just as dangerous as intercourse, so don't think that you're safe with your hot new guy because there's no penetration happening (see Principle #5). Some sexually transmitted diseases are incurable—once you have one, you can't give it back. Besides, are you really going to enjoy having sex with a guy when you have a feeling he's putting you at risk?

Empowering Reason: Problem-Spotting

What to Say: "Hmm, did it always look that way, babe?"

If an issue arises down the line in your relationship, like a strange bump or discharge, you'll notice it and be able to bring it to your man's attention. But only if you were paying attention from jump street. That means you're not just interested in getting a good look at his penis the first time you two fool around. You're interested in taking a good look on a regular basis so you can spot changes.

As a Mrs. and an MD, I'm well aware that it's easier to get a man to stop the car and ask for directions than it is to get him to stop what he's doing and go to the doctor (but both are pretty difficult). One study showed that 31 percent of men delayed getting treated or tested for STIs for more than a week—and up to several months—putting them at risk for additional infections and potentially even infertility. We women are used to planting our feet into stirrups at least once a year, whereas men book an appointment to see their physician about as frequently as they buy tickets to go to a Broadway show. But that doesn't mean that we ladies should quit trying to get them to go . . . to both.

Empowering Reason: Praise

What to Say: "Baby, it's the biggest I've ever seen."

You've got to see what he's working with so you can pay him a genuine compliment. You might have the most beautiful penis in the world in the palm of your hand, but if you're not taking a peek at it, you'll never know. By the way, whether or not it's the biggest or the most beautiful, there is other ego-boosting admiration to be offered to his King P. It might be thick—just the way you like 'em—hard as a rock, or full of (pleasurable) surprises. Some men are growers not showers, meaning their flaccid penis is much smaller than their erect penis. Look away and you'll miss the boom and bust.

Empowering Reason: Pleasure

What to Say: "Boo, I know exactly what I want to do with that."

Every penis is a little different. Some are short while others stretch on for inches. Some are tapered while others are thick through and through. My Notorious V.A.G.s might be experienced enough to take one look at their man's hard-on, grab him by the penis, and lead him to the bedroom knowing exactly how to get their ooh-ooh-ooh. But the rest of us might have to do some research on the internet or phone a friend.

Once you've gotten a good look or feel, you can figure out how his Jack can bring your Jill a whole lot more pleasure. Did you know the average penis length is five to seven inches when hard? If he's less gifted in the length department, you might want to try positions that allow maximum deep penetration, like doggie style with a deep curve in your back or reverse cowgirl with a pillow under his butt. If he's more extraordinarily gifted (yes, you can have too much of a good thing), you might try positions that keep the level of penetration in *your* control, like cowgirl or facing each other on your side.

Empowering Reason: Pride

What to Say: "Things are starting to look up for me!"

So many women have trouble maintaining eye contact with other people, much less a lingering stare at a man's penis. Please know that I'm talking about in person—not that NSFW (not safe for work), racy Instagram pic your bestie sent you. My Virgin Marys and Sanctified Snatches in particular need to be proud they stared down the one-eyed monster. You'll find there was nothing to be frightened by in the first place. In fact, it's kind of cute.

CHARTING YOUR COURSE TO HIS NETHERLANDS

When it comes to vacations, there are two kinds of people in this world: improvisers and planners. Improvisers don't look before they leap. They are like college kids who go on spring break trips without any sense of what's in store. Their suitcase is packed (condoms? check!) and they're ready for fun in the sun in Cancun (sunscreen? check!). However, if you ask them the name of the hotel where they're staying, they just stare back at you and blink. (By the way, you don't have to be young, dumb, and full of watered-down rum to do a vacation on the fly. There are plenty of grown-and-flown free spirits who prefer spontaneous trips to up the excitement level of their time off.)

Then there are the planners. People who like to map out every single day of their trip—even if that only means knowing that they'll be lying by the beach on Monday, lying by the pool on Tuesday, back to the beach on Wednesday . . . well, you get the idea.

Here's what I want you to remember: if you're taking a trip to your man's Netherlands, there's no room for improvisation. Be a planner for that excursion rather than just seeing what pops up once you arrive. Be prepared to use all your senses on this journey—just like you would on any vacation. You should expect to take in all the sights, sounds, scents, and feels of this new locale you're about to (literally) uncover. Here's how:

Listen to What Locals Say

And by "locals," I mean your man. Have you noticed that he's been complaining about his member at all lately? Has he been letting out some "ow!"s when he uses your bathroom? Scratching his crotch more aggressively than usual? All of these could be signs that he has an infection or an infestation (like crabs).

Take in the Scents

Let's be honest, your man's crotch isn't going to smell like a field of roses—but it shouldn't smell like a fish market either. The next time you're lying in your man's lap or after you've kissed your way down his chest, be sure to catch a whiff of what's coming from his pants. Just as with women, a foul smell (along with a yellowish discharge) could be gonorrhea in men.

Plan a Feel Trip Before Your Field Trip

Welcome to the part of the journey where things really start to get interesting. You're about to let your hands give you some information your ears and nose can't. A few years ago, a Mary Jane came to me for her routine physical but ended up spilling the details of her latest feel trip. "I've got damaged goods, Dr. Jackie," MJ revealed after a disappointing dry-humping session with her new boo. "When I put my hand down his boxers, I could feel that his penis curved to the right. Hard." She pointed her index finger at me and then curled it down so it looked like a hook. Ladies, meet Peyronie's disease.

Don't worry, you can't catch it. It's basically what happens when scar tissue forms inside the penis, making it curve in a particular direction. Experts aren't sure what causes Peyronie's, but they do believe repeated injury to the penis (perhaps during sports) can have an impact. Up to 23 percent of men between forty and seventy have the ailment, so as you get older you're more likely to encounter a sexual partner with it.

My MJ client wanted to know one thing and one thing alone: "Does it still work?" She was using her feel trip for empowerment in the pleasure zone. She had the right question but the wrong expert. MJ needed to be talking to her boo. Depending on how severe the curve is, some men do experience difficulty having sex or maintaining an erection. But it depends on the man and how sharp the curve is. MJ could've benefited from a few Google searches too. If your man has a curved penis, depending on which way it bends, there are positions you might try that could actually rock your world. (If it bends up, you might want to try spooning sex, 69, or a pogo-stick position where you're both upright but your legs are wrapped around his waist and your arms are around his chest.)

Besides pleasure, a feel trip can also empower you through prevention. While you're rubbing, stroking, or squeezing his member, you want to see if you feel any patches of small rough bumps that feel like a head of cauliflower in texture. Those could be genital warts caused by HPV.

If you feel what could be small blisters (they might be pus-filled or crusty) or sores, this could be herpes and you'll need to be very careful. The blisters can be highly contagious, so you'll want to stop your feel trip and thoroughly wash your hands before touching anything else. Herpes can be transmitted to any other part of your body, including your eyes, mouth, and genitals. It can also infect broken skin. So if you were to touch a sore and then scratch your leg, you could have an outbreak there if the skin were cut.

A quick reminder: if your man's uncircumcised, it is best to rub him in a way that pulls back that foreskin so you can see his whole penis.

Go Sightseeing

This is the part where you take a long, hard look at your man's penis. The most important thing to remember is that you need to leave the lights on! Whether you make it fun ("This means you get to see me with the lights on too, boo!"), romantic ("I want to see every incredibly sexy inch of you"), or flat-out honest ("So, I have this policy before I have sex with someone"), please don't even dim the lights. You could also try doing this while taking a shower with your man, which could give you a longer look and better feel.

Just like with the feel trip, when you're sightseeing you want to check for any bumps. With herpes and HPV they can be flesh-colored or whitish. You should also be on the lookout for anything that moves. That's right, your eyes aren't fooling you. Crabs (pubic lice) are big enough for you to spot with your naked eye and they're easily spread. Finally, be on the lookout for discharge that doesn't look like pre-ejaculate or ejaculate. Gonorrhea, for example, can produce a white, yellow, or greenish discharge from the penis.

You'll notice that I didn't mention one sense: taste. That's because I don't want you putting anything in your mouth that hasn't been inspected or tested. It's not uncommon for infections like gonorrhea, syphilis, HPV, and others to be transmitted orally.

If at any point on this planned excursion you notice that something is odd about his penis, don't ignore your intuition. End the trip early.

POINT OF V: INSPECT EVERY INCH

One of my Notorious V.A.G. patients once told me about a professional athlete she dated who was worth millions. Handsome? You bet. Fairy-tale dates? Definitely, girl. A real sweetheart at times? Mm-hmm. But she dumped him—because his penis was too small. In sports they say that winning isn't everything, it's the only thing. Well, with sex I want to flip that script. Size isn't everything, it's just one thing. So many women I know will talk about feeling their man up to get a sense how big it is. I want women taking that feel trip to figure out how healthy their man is— not how hung he is.

While checking out your man's member is important, it's really only about 10 percent of what you should be doing to protect your Queen V. If you're planning on having unprotected sex, you and your partner should both get tested for sexually transmitted infections. You've also got to sit down and have serious conversations with your partner about safe sex, exposure to infections, and monogamy (see Principle #5). Kings and queens rule their kingdom together. You need to look out for each other so you can both have long, healthy reigns.

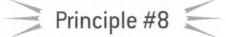

Principle #8

Know When to Leave
Sex Toys to the Professionals

HOW COULD SHE NOT FEEL ANY NUTS?

A few years ago, an embarrassed Mary Jane came into my office after a week of wearing pads when it wasn't her period. She wouldn't let anyone—except me—get within whiffing distance of her Queen V thanks to a mysterious, smelly brown discharge that had been coming out of her for days. It didn't itch and it wasn't painful. But it was making her feel so unpretty.

My first thought was that Mary Jane had wiped—or did something else—from back to front. I was expecting an infection at best and rectal incontinence at worst. Once she was in the stirrups, I put the speculum in place, and all I can say is that it was a *hot mess* inside her. Besides the overwhelming smell, her vagina looked like it had chunks of dried blood swirled together with a sticky mucus. I went in expecting to see stool, but this was . . . something different.

"Have you changed your bathing routine lately?" I asked her. "Have you been doing anything different down here?"

"No, nothing I can think of," she said.

Part of any exam is what I can detect as a doctor. But the other part is what you tell me as a patient. And I need my patients to give me all the information they can. Unfortunately, a lot of women dance around the truth until I'm getting ready to leave the room. (Don't make me work so hard, ladies! I'm here for you and your Queen V—and I'm not judging you.)

Those who aren't dancing are genuinely forgetful. Either way it's worth a repeat ask. So I tried her once more while I started removing chunks of whatever I was looking at out of her vagina.

"Are you sure?" I said again. "You can't think of anything different you might've put in here?" When it suddenly hit her, she almost sat all the way up on the table.

"He's a big dummy!" she yelled. "If he messed me up, I don't know what I'll do." Then she started giving me the whole story she'd forgotten of how her boyfriend had stuck fun-size candy bars in (and out and in) her as part of foreplay a week ago. Apparently, there is something two sticks of Twix can't fix. Well, to be accurate, it was a Snickers. And since no candy bar left behind wasn't her man's motto, she ended up with a mashed-up, mushed-up mess of chocolate and peanuts oozing out of her vagina. "How could she not feel any nuts?" I thought to myself.

"This is all his fault!" she said. But really, it takes two to turn your Queen V into a candy aisle at a convenience store with no AC in the middle of summer, right? I cleaned her out, put her on antibiotics, and reminded her that our Queen Vs don't have a sweet tooth.

You might be thinking that I'm sharing this story because it goes against everything I believe in regarding protecting your Queen V's health—and excessive intake of sweets. Or because I'm a little miffed that women tend to get the short end of the stick. (Why exactly did her man opt for fun size instead of king size?) But I'm actually trying to drive home a completely different point for your Queen V's health: instead of getting inventive on your way to better sex, leave creating sex toys to the professionals so you can stay out of the exam room.

WHAT EVERY GROWN WOMAN CAN GAIN FROM A TOY COLLECTION

Before I lose my Virgin Marys, Sanctified Snatches, and Coochie-Chondriacs (who I'm sure were just floored by that sexual chocolate catastrophe), let me ask you a quick question. What do a feather, a pillow, a blindfold, and a four-inch foam platform have in common? They're all considered erotic toys. That's right. The category isn't just about dildos and vibrators. So for my VPs on the more reserved end of the spectrum, don't shut down immediately while this chapter delves into mastering all your sexual possibilities. Just like you, toys run the spectrum from quietly tantalizing to out-of-this-world excitement. But first, let's talk about why you would want to use a sex toy in the first place.

1. You Want to Orgasm in Under Thirty Seconds

Yup, there's a toy for that. They're called clitoral suckers and women are raving about them. But if you just want to have better sex—off the clock—toys can help. Plenty of women have difficulty achieving arousal, perhaps because they're going through menopause or another health condition. The right toys and lubricants can work wonders for increased clitoral stimulation, greater blood flow, and overcoming dryness.

2. You Want to Get Closer to Your Partner

Didn't see that one coming, did you? Yes, you can use toys alone, but you can also use them with your boyfriend, girlfriend, or spouse to enhance your sexual experience—not point out inadequacies. Some women have difficulty orgasming while their husband or boyfriend is inside them. (At least a third of women require clitoral stimulation to climax, with another third saying that it makes their orgasm better.) Toys like vibrators can help you climax together. Lesbian partners might want to introduce a penis into the mix without having a male in the room. Long-distance couples can enjoy toys that are controlled by Wi-Fi. So if you're in Georgia and your partner's in California, they can still have a hand (literally) in turning you on without being in the same room. Some people refer to these toys as "teledildonics."

3. You Want to Get to Know Your Body Better

You have to know what you like in order to be able to tell someone else. Or, better yet, show someone else. Maybe you need a little help finding your G-spot and a vibrator geared specifically toward stimulating it can help you have that ooh-ooh-ooh breakthrough. Or you're curious about butt plugs but don't trust someone else to explore that with you. Here's your, um, way in.

4. You Could Use Some Support

The sex toy category includes pillows, cushions, wedges, and furniture items that can support your body, help you open your legs wider, or hold positions longer. If you've ever worried about having the flexibility, mobility, or energy to get it on, the right toy might be able to help.

5. You're Curious About Hotter Sex

Erotic toys let you step outside your comfort zone—almost all the way out—but still stay in the realm of being safe. You can role-play and live out your wildest fantasies (a threesome? Sex with a woman? French maid?) while never having to worry about any real-life repercussions. How's that for letting your freak flag fly?

SEXUAL ANATOMY 102: YOUR G-SPOT AND BEYOND

If sex toys have taught us anything, it's that there's more than one way to stroke a cat. Whether your partner flutters a feather across the back of your neck or the lips of your labia, it sends a message to your brain that things are about to get pretty exciting. Back in Principle #1, we covered external anatomy to get you familiar with your flower, and in Principle #11, we'll talk about reproductive anatomy to explain what parts of your body help with making a baby. Here's where we'll cover pure pleasure. Meet the places your Queen V craves to be touched.

- **clitoris.** It has one job and one job alone: to bring you pleasure. Greek for the word "key," it can open the door to an amazing evening (or morning or afternoon).
- **G-spot.** After years of experts saying it was a myth, a recent study confirmed the existence of this sensual zone inside your vagina. It's a small, spongy spot located about a third of the way inside your vaginal canal on the belly side. If you were to insert your finger inside your Queen V and make a tickle or come-hither motion, you'd have a good chance of stimulating it.
- **perineum.** This thin stretch of tissue going from your vaginal canal to your anal canal can be oh-so-sensitive to the touch.
- **anus.** If you're open to a way out being a way in, backdoor play can be extremely stimulating due to all the nerve endings in the area, even taking you straight over the edge into orgasm.

THE VP OF SEX TOYS

Sex sells . . . and apparently sex toys sell much better. Erotic items are a $24 billion (that's right, with a B) industry that has entered a new stratosphere of capabilities in recent years. I've seen gold-plated vibrators that cost more than a car and saddle-style sex machines you ride like a cowgirl for the cost of a vacation in Paris. Adult toys come in every eye-popping size, porn-star-inspired shape, and irresistible color you can imagine. They can warm up to body temperature, thrust in and out, and simulate the feel of human skin on their coital quest to get you faster orgasms, closer connection with your partner, or deeper penetration.

So if you're feeling adventurous, how do you know which one's right for you? Decide according to your VP. Follow these suggestions from my friends Kandi Burruss, a certified sex coach and owner of the award-winning Bedroom Kandi toy line, and Angela Lieben, director of marketing and communications for Liberator, an Atlanta-based company that designs sex furniture and sells pleasure objects worldwide online.

If You're a Virgin Mary . . .

Rest assured that you can start your exploration with toys that are so discreet no one would know what they were—even if they found them sitting out on your dining room table. These days, vibrators come in the tiniest of packages that look like lipstick cases or compacts. That means you get to experiment with getting your jollies without having your feathers ruffled by an all-too-intimidating toy. You could also look for pleasure things that encourage a more hands-on experience, like small vibrators that attach to your fingers so they feel more like a part of you. If you're bold enough to head into a shop (clearly at an odd hour when it's likely to be empty), be brave and ask for help finding something entry-level. If you're searching online shops, try looking for "discreet," "travel-size," and "quiet" items.

If You're a Sanctified Snatch . . .

You probably still want to camouflage any gear for getting off. Since you think of sex more for procreation than recreation, try looking into toys that could help you boost your bedroom confidence and feel connected to yourself. You might be more comfortable with items that help you enhance your experience with your partner, like a revealing bra or a small vibrator you can use while your partner is inside you. If you're searching online shops, try looking for "couples toys," "lingerie," and "discreet" toys.

If You're a Coochie-Chondriac . . .

What you care most about is hygiene so you can stop stressing about whether or not the toy could be harming you and start climaxing. Once you find a toy you like, check the product description or packaging to see if it's hypoallergenic, nonporous (meaning that it won't hold on to bacteria or be hard to clean), and latex-free, in case you're concerned about allergies. Materials you want to look for: medical-grade silicone, Pyrex, or stainless steel. What you may want to avoid: vinyl, PVC, rubber, and jelly—all materials that tend to contain phthalates (chemicals that have been linked to health concerns like breast cancer, obesity, and others). Or take the opposite approach and only shop from companies that carry natural products, like Chakrubs, Njoy, and Organic Loven.

If You're a Mary Jane . . .

This isn't your first rodeo. You're bold enough to walk into a shop and poke around until you find something you like, and you've probably already had at least one toy in your dresser drawer before. So think about upgrading. If you're in a store, let them know what you've liked in the past and ask what the next generation of that is. Maybe you want to level up from your old vibrator to one that's shaped like a tongue or that targets your G-spot. Or you want something that's waterproof so you can experiment in the bath. Sex toys are also a great way for this VP to try a sexual scenarios that she'd never live out in real life. If you (or your partner) have ever fantasized about a threesome or wanted to pretend to be a quarterback and a cheerleader behind the bleachers, now's your chance. If you're searching online shops, try "best sellers" or "costumes."

If You're a Notorious V.A.G. . . .

You don't need my help going buck wild. You already know that toys are your gateway to experiences most people have never imagined and would need a three-hour PowerPoint presentation to figure out. For you, pleasure objects help you take sex to the next level by wearing a double-ended strapless strap-on or lying back on a sex chaise for deeper penetration. As an early erotic adopter, you're trying out that sex swing or Wi-Fi-enabled vibrator as soon as it hits the shelves. You're also voted girl most likely to get something for your partner. How thoughtful—for both of you. If you're searching online shops, try "new arrivals," "tech," "for him," and "furniture."

DON'T FORGET TO CLEAN UP AFTER CLIMAX

Back in Principles #5 and 8, I gave you a rundown of how to clean your sex toys. Let me say it again, this is important—even though we know there are folks out there who never do it at all. Follow the cleaning and storage instructions in the booklet your toy came with or consider buying a storage box that doubles as an ultraviolet cleaner to make things easy on yourself.

THE SPECIALIST'S CORNER: PLEASURE OBJECTS

Whether you think dildos are a dil-don't or you have a secret closet in your home that could double as a sex shop, you're going to want to read all the sexual goodies Angela Lieben shared during our "V" Q&A. As the director of marketing and communications for Liberator, an Atlanta-based company that designs sex furniture and sells pleasure objects worldwide online, she tests out sex toys before they hit the shelf and writes about them on the company blog. (And her readers have never been more thankful for a woman willing to kiss and tell.) Here's what she revealed about how much money to spend on a toy, what to do if you're worried about getting addicted to your vibrator, and the very best sex toy ever.

Dr. Jackie: Walking into a sex shop or going to one online can make a girl feel like a kid in a candy store—but it's a candy store where a lot of us have no idea what the flavors are. How can women figure out what sex toy to try?

> Lieben: Ask yourself if you're interested in external, internal, or
> dual stimulation. External stimulation would be objects that
> are non-insertable and meant for arousing the clitoris or other

erogenous zones like the nipples. Internal stimulation means your vagina or the anus. Then there are dual-stimulation products that do both!

Dr. Jackie: Once you decide which category you want to explore, what's next?

Lieben: Think about whether you want vibration—so a product that needs to be charged or run on batteries—or no vibration—like a dildo. If you're in a store, don't be afraid to touch an item. I actually tell women to try out vibrators in store by turning them on and putting them on the tip of their nose because I think the nose is like the clitoris of the face. It's very sensitive, so you can kind of get a sense of what that object would feel like. Also, if you can find them, read online reviews.

Dr. Jackie: So let's say you find something but you have sticker shock. Some of these toys cost a pretty penny.

Lieben: I like to think of pleasure objects like a good pair of shoes: they can look beautiful and feel great, but you have to invest in them. Our bodies are designed for pleasure. We deserve a pleasurable sex life. Keep that in mind as you set a budget for yourself first, and then look at products in that range.

Dr. Jackie: Now, I've heard stories about people finding their battery-powered soul mate and getting addicted to it. What's your take?

Lieben: I wouldn't say addicted, but they may rely on it too much. If you begin to rely too much on your object, I would say switch things up. Start using your hands or a different toy—if you've been using something external, switch to an internal object. We're habit-forming creatures, so it's going to be more of a habit than an addiction. But honestly, nothing can ever replace the feeling of your partner.

Dr. Jackie: Speaking of partners, how do you get them on board with a sex toy?

Lieben: That's one of the biggest questions I get. You always want to have a conversation with your partner outside the bedroom to express your desires. Maybe bring an article that you read in a magazine or book and say, 'Hey, honey, I just read that Beyoncé dropped a lot of money in a sex toy shop" or "Eva Longoria is talking about sex toys. Want to give them a try?" Once you get past that step, shop together. You can do it online or in a store.

Dr. Jackie: What if you have a toy because you have used it before and you want to introduce it into the relationship?

Lieben: Never whip it out during the heat of the moment. I would just say "I'd like to introduce you to a little friend of mine" or "This makes me feel good, do you want to watch me use it?" People are voyeurs, they like to watch. Give them the opportunity to see what makes you feel good. Maybe use it a couple of times and then find something new that you both can use together. Watch out though: one guy I dated was adamant that he was going to keep our sex toys after the breakup because he didn't want me using them with somebody else.

Dr. Jackie: Last question: I've got to know what you consider to be the best sex toy ever.

Lieben: It's the same for everyone: your own hands. They never run out of batteries and you feel absolutely everything.

POINT OF V: GO WITH THE PROS

Once I saw a couple in the ER who were so embarrassed by what had happened to them, they kept tossing the responsibility for explaining it to me back and forth like a ping-pong ball.

"Are you going to tell her what happened?" the husband said to his Mary Jane wife.

"Um, no. I think you should," she replied.

"Actually, I think you should," he said.

I let them go in circles for about a minute before I finally said, "Well, somebody better say something soon."

And they did. She had a flower vase stuck inside her. The suction at the mouth of the container was so tight that it wouldn't release its grip on her cervix. They couldn't get it out so they had to (carefully) make their way to the emergency room with the hope that a doctor could do the trick. I can't take credit for freeing this woman from a flower vase. I had to pull in a colleague who was able to maneuver it out of her. But I think you get the picture. Whether it's a desire to be adventurous or a level of embarrassment that keeps you from ordering something online, I want to get you away from household items and into the hands of professionals. That'll keep you in the bedroom and out of the emergency room.

Treat Your Period Like a Frenemy

"WE WERE FRIENDLY . . . BUT I COULD'VE PUSHED HER DOWN THE STAIRS AND NOT FELT BAD."

Anyone who has ever watched pledges walk in lockstep across a yard or seen them dressed up in strange costumes during a Chemistry 101 class knows that people join Greek life to basically bond with and become a part of a new family. Sorority sisters are supposed to behave as *sisters* do. And oh boy, did we! When I became an Alpha Kappa Alpha in college, I adored all my sisters. But I have to admit that I had a seriously competitive relationship with one of them.

This soror and I were both science majors and constantly vying for the best grades in our classes. We were cordial out loud, but you wouldn't believe how I cut her down in my head. When I saw her, I'd be kind enough to tell her, "You look good today!" But in my mind, I was thinking, "Don't slip and fall on anything, girlfriend." We had so much fakery going on that it would make you nauseous to hear us complimenting the other.

We were both into fashion, had great taste in clothes, and dressed well. However, she was one hot mama who could regularly outdress me in her head-to-toe neon outfits or suits with shoulder pads big enough to take out a quarterback. (This was the '80s, remember?) It drove me crazy. I could've pushed her down the stairs and not felt bad if she got bruised. Bye, Felicia! Why? It was basically for one reason and one reason alone: we liked the same really handsome guy.

Now I know you're not used to hearing me talk like this. That's not the kind, consoling, peacekeeping Dr. Jackie you know and love. But I'm speaking a truth from my past. And I know I'm not alone. We've all had these kinds of rivalries in our lives at some point. Whether it's a coworker gunning for the same promotion you are or an annoying sibling trying to get more of your parents' attention, I'm positive every woman can think of someone that she's had a frenemy-type relationship with. If you can't think of someone who was one-part friend, one-part enemy, I'm about to introduce you to her now: meet your period.

WHAT IS A PERIOD?

Simply put, your period is a two-to-seven-day stretch of time in which the endometrial lining of your uterus is shed and comes out through your vagina. It's triggered by hormones that start in your brain and happens every twenty-one to thirty-five days. Afterward, it leaves behind a fresh lining of your uterus that waits for you to get pregnant. That lining is the healthy tissue and fertile soil needed for implantation. If you don't become pregnant, the cycle starts over again. If you do, you head down a completely different forty-week path.

That's the simple physical definition. The problem is, checking into the Red Roof Inn (meaning your period) for the first time is a much more emotionally complex experience. Initially, you either love it or you hate it. Your first period can be a beautiful rite of passage where your mother holds an elaborate "First Moon Party" or "Period Party" for you, like Tyra Banks's mom did. But it could also be a dreaded event that makes you want to knock that red-and-white "Congrats on Your Period!" cake right off the counter and onto the floor. Periods can be a cause for joy and celebration because some cultures like to say it signifies womanhood. But they can also be messy, painful causes of sadness because your dad and your brother won't roughhouse with you anymore. If you're a transgender woman, hearing other women rip open a plastic tampon package may be a difficult reminder of something you'll never experience. And if you're a transgender man who menstruates, your period could be a difficult reminder of something you desperately want to get rid of.

Once you accept calling a Code Red a recurring part of your life, you and your period will become best frenemies. Just like any frenemy, dealing with her is emotionally draining and can make you want to cut ties—perhaps by taking continuous contraceptives or getting a hysterectomy. She knows exactly how to mortify you in public, like on those days your tampon string slips out of your bathing suit or you're wearing white pants . . . with a red dot. And that chick undercuts your performance at work with distracting headaches and cramps. You're ecstatic and relieved to see her after you've had a condom break on you (phew!). You're enraged or depressed when she pops up after you've been trying for months to get pregnant (damn, damn, damn!).

It's easy to feel overwhelmed when dealing with a frenemy. Sometimes you might just want to give in. "All right, I guess I'm not going to work today," you'll say. "Fine, no sex. You win," you might think. But, ladies. Never take the crown off your Queen V. Instead, nestle it on your head nice and tight because you're getting ready to surf the crimson tide like an Olympic athlete.

THE SUBTLE ART OF BESTING A FRENEMY

No need to reinvent the wheel here. The exact same strategies that women use for dealing with frenemies who come around at school and work can be used for dealing with the frenemy that comes around for leak week. Master these techniques and your period will never be the boss of you again. You are the queen. Not your period:

Maintain close tabs on that chick. Eliminate the element of surprise by
staying on top of where she is at all times. She can't surprise you by
dropping in uninvited on a romantic date if you're tracking her like
an FBI agent about to make a bust (see "How to Track Your Cycle
and What It All Means" on page 155). It doesn't have to be a lot
of pencil-and-paper work. There are dozens of period tracker apps
(like Clue, Flo, and Glow) that are free, easy to use, and give you a
heads-up when you're approaching a red light. They'll also let you
make note of your symptoms so you start to notice if you're hornier

than usual right before she arrives or if you tend to have your worst cramps on the first day she shows up. Once you can anticipate her moves, you'll be able to stay one step ahead of her by planning your Caribbean vacation around her or simply keeping your supply of Advil up. Tracking can also help you notice if something's wrong and it's time to talk to your doctor, like your period has gone missing (amenorrhea) or your cramps (dysmenorrhea) are a 10 on a scale of 1 to 10 (perhaps indicating endometriosis).

Keep calm and carry backup. When a real-life frenemy catches you off guard, it helps to have a quick clapback or a good friend at your side to jump in and help you out. When your period catches you off guard, all you need is an extra tampon or pad in your purse so you're never at Aunt Flo's mercy. If not for yourself, then for your friend or coworker who finds herself in a pinch and needs to "borrow" a tampon. Having the right backup tools is everything.

Some experts believe you can sync up and get on the same cycle as other women you spend a lot of time around just by proximity. So you and your sister might be at risk for a surprise visit at the same time of the month. New research is debunking the idea, but anecdotally it's still going strong. I once had a mother and a daughter—in separate exam rooms—in my office at the same time on the same cycle. "Put them on some mood stabilizers, get them on birth control, or take them to your house, Dr. Jackie," the husband/father pleaded with me. That poor man was going out of his mind every month making trips to the drugstore for them to pick up tampons (but then realizing he should've bought pads) and getting yelled at when he got home. They were running him ragged and he was getting it from both sides.

Feel free to refuse her invitations. Even with people we love, we have to set boundaries. That goes double for your period. So if your frenemy asks about having a party at your "pad" and you'd rather not this month, just say no. You can skip a period altogether by using continuous contraception (like Seasonique birth control pills or skipping the hormone-free week with pills, the patch, and the ring). Up to 20 percent of women who have hormonal IUDs put in stop getting their period entirely. If you're completely through with the relationship, you can get rid of your periods through surgery (such as endometrial ablation).

Don't believe her lies. It's tempting to believe what your red frenemy is telling you by showing up, disappearing, or waltzing in late, but don't. She can be oh-so-deceptive.

- A period is typically an indication that a woman has ovulated and didn't get pregnant. But women who are pregnant sometimes do get a period.
- Just because you're late or missed a period doesn't mean you're pregnant. (You could be stressed, exercising too much, or have a thyroid problem.)
- A period gone missing doesn't mean you're in menopause. (You need to miss twelve in a row for that to happen.)
- Just because you're getting a period doesn't mean getting pregnant will be easy.

Don't put your faith in your frenemy. If you're trying to get pregnant, worried about missing periods, or concerned about entering menopause, give your OB-GYN a heads-up and ask her for advice you can trust (and see Principle #11 on fertility).

Know what she's capable of. I don't mean to scare you, but I've seen blood flow from a woman's vagina like a faucet was turned on. While your period can help you bring life into this world, she can take life away as well. Always have a sense of how light or (more importantly) how heavy your flow is so you can notice a problem. If you need to change pads in the middle of the night or are bleeding for more than a week, that's a sign something may be wrong and you need to escalate this encounter by meeting with your OB-GYN (see "Abnormal Bleeding" on page 160).

Let the rivalry motivate you. Yes, frenemies can be a thorn in your side. But they can also be a good thing. Every woman needs to have someone in her life who keeps her on her toes. Your frenemy can do just that. Allow your period to inspire you to get to know your body better, pay closer attention to your health, and maximize your well-being.

HOW TO TRACK YOUR CYCLE AND WHAT IT ALL MEANS

If anyone is the boss of your Queen V (yes, the hierarchy goes higher) it would be hormones. Estrogen, progesterone, luteinizing hormone, and other hormones control what she does, when she does it, and how she feels while doing it. Hormones are also the key players when it comes to your menstrual cycle, triggering the release of eggs, the thickening of your uterine wall, and other functions. Here's a quick rundown of what to expect in the four different phases of your cycle.

Menstrual Phase

Your first full day of flow is Day 1 of your cycle. On average, this phase lasts from three days up to a week as your body sheds a combination of blood, tissue, and mucus from your uterus when no implantation of an embryo has taken place. You'll release anywhere from two to four tablespoons of menstrual fluid over the course of this phase. An average pad or tampon can hold about one ounce.

Follicular Phase

This phase overlaps with your period but continues for longer. Follicle-stimulating hormone prompts your ovaries to prepare multiple follicles to release an egg. But only one or two (making it possible for you to have fraternal twins) will make the journey in the end. This preparation phase lasts for about two weeks.

Ovulatory Phase

In the shortest phase of them all—it lasts between sixteen and thirty-two hours—an egg is released. It makes its journey from the ovary down through the fallopian tube (where fertilization takes place) to wait for sperm. Some women experience pain (called mittelschmerz) for a few minutes to a few hours when the egg departs. It's pain small enough to nag you but not severe enough to cause you to be doubled over. It occurs because once the egg is released, follicular fluid irritates the abdominal lining. There's an upside to ovulation as well. Research shows women may get a little spike in their libido around that time. It may be your body's way of encouraging you to have sex and make a baby.

All of this happens around Day 14 if you're on a 28-day cycle. If you're tracking your progress in order to get pregnant, this is the most important point for you to take note of. You may see an increase in cervical mucus or an ever-so-slight rise in your basal body temperature (taken first thing in the morning before you get out of bed) at ovulation. Those are your key signs.

Luteal Phase

During this two-week phase, your body awaits implantation, maintaining a thick uterine lining for the embryo. Whether you're pregnant or not, you may experience breast tenderness, fatigue, and bloating. This could be PMS or just early signs that you're pregnant. Sometimes it's hard to tell.

PERIODS GONE WRONG

One of my Notorious V.A.G. patients had her period come for her. Hard. At work. This Notorious V.A.G. had a very strong personality in every way: she's very confident, independent, and strong-willed—perhaps a little overbearing. That was fine and dandy three weeks out of the month. But a week before her period would arrive, things went haywire.

She'd have complete and total meltdowns at her job, getting so angry at times that she'd curse at her coworkers when they made mistakes on projects and publicly yell at her subordinates when they took too long to reply to her emails. Her boss warned her about her verbal outbursts several times, but in the heat of those bad weeks, she'd say, "I don't care. Fire me!" So they eventually did. She ended up in my office a few days before her insurance ran out.

Ladies, I want you coming to me before things go south. Don't wait until you wake up, say uh-oh, and it's too late to fix the situation. When you realize after keeping tabs on your period that there seems to be a pattern to things going wrong, come talk to me so we can figure out a solution. Whether you're suffering from premenstrual dysmorphic disorder (PMDD), like this woman was, or something else, we can usually help. Here are the most common ways your frenemy can mess you up—and what to do about it.

Premenstrual Dysmorphic Disorder (PMDD)

What it is: While as many as 80 percent of menstruating women experience PMS, up to 8 percent of menstruating women go through a much more severe form called PMDD. This is not the normal moodiness, anxiety, or feeling a little down that can throw a wrench in your attitude the week before your period. It's a lot more intense and it inhibits your ability to function normally—like my Notorious V.A.G. patient who just couldn't pull it together at her job. Think: anger, depression, lack of control, and insomnia. There are also physical symptoms like breast tenderness, weight gain, acne, and headaches.

My running joke is that you can't have PMDD every day of the month. If you do, that's B.I.T.C.H.Y. There's a beginning and an end when it comes to PMDD. And if that week of the month destroys your ability to maintain a relationship, your marriage, or your job, then it's a problem you really need to talk to your doctor about.

Why it happens: We're not really sure. It may be that you're more sensitive to the hormonal changes that occur with your menstrual cycle or it could be linked to low levels of serotonin, a chemical in the brain tied to controlling mood. Having a personal or family history of PMS, PMDD, depression, or other mood disorders can increase your likelihood of having PMDD.

How to treat it: First things first, tag a friend who can give you a heads-up when your symptoms arise. I've been told by patients with PMDD that they don't even realize when it's happening to them. Authorize a good friend at work or home to put her arm around you and check in if your attitude seems to have gone off the rails. She can gently say, "You were a little rough on Jill today. Any chance you're dealing with PMDD this week?" Let her know you won't strike out at her and that you'll appreciate her looking out for you.

Then talk to your doctor about your options. I tell my PMDD patients to change their lifestyle habits as a first line of defense. Eat whole foods, get more fruits and vegetables in your diet, eliminate sweets and salts, exercise more, take a multivitamin, and make sure you're getting enough magnesium (which would be somewhere between 310 mg and 400 mg per day for adult women depending upon your age and pregnancy status). You might also consider hormonal contraceptives specifically shown to treat PMDD, period elimination (by taking continuous contraceptives), antidepressants, and behavior modification (like stress-management techniques).

Menstrual Migraine

What it is: A severe headache that occurs in the two days before or the first three days of your period.

Why it happens: Hormonal fluctuations, particularly the drop in estrogen just before your period.

How to treat it: Your doctor will choose one of three different strategies for eliminating or lessening the intensity of these headaches, depending upon their frequency and severity. These include continuous contraception (perhaps taking a break every three to six months), medication taken days before your period to prevent the onset of a migraine (including low-estrogen birth control pills so there's less of a drop in estrogen), and medication used to treat the migraine once it arrives (like tryptophan, which can stop migraine pain).

Dysmenorrhea (Menstrual Pain)

What it is: Killer cramps. Primary dysmenorrhea occurs when, just before or at the beginning of their period, women feel sharp spasms of pain in their lower abdomen that can last a few days. Alternately, you might feel a dull ache in your pelvis, lower back, hips, and inner thighs. I see scared young girls all the time with cramping so bad it's debilitating. They can't function and my heart goes out to them. I just want to shield them from that pain. Depending upon the severity, up to 90% of women are affected by dysmenorrhea during their period.

Secondary dysmenorrhea is period pain tied to another health concern like PID, endometriosis, fibroids, or adenomyosis (see Principle #12).

Why it happens: The physical symptoms of primary dysmenorrhea have been tied to the uterus contracting in order to push out menstrual blood. Levels of a troublemaking hormone called prostaglandin, made in the lining of your uterus, increase leading up to and peak on the first day of your period. Prostaglandin triggers the contractions.

How to treat it: Nonsteroidal anti-inflammatory drugs (NSAIDs) work best for relieving pain linked to primary dysmenorrhea and prostaglandin fluctuations. I also offer my patients hormonal birth control options to alleviate the pain. We're not really trying to control birth so much as we're manipulating the hormonal spikes to avoid killer cramping. If you have secondary dysmenorrhea, talk to your doctor about treating the specific cause of your pain, which may require outpatient surgery.

Lifestyle changes and natural remedies may have an impact

on lessening your cramps as well, according to some small studies. Aerobic exercise or just stretching three days a week; adopting a low-fat vegetarian diet; fish oil and vitamin B1 supplements; acupuncture and even massaging essential oils on the lower abdomen have been tied to reduced period pain.

Abnormal Bleeding

What it is: It's as broad as is sounds. Abnormal bleeding is anything that falls outside the normal range of menstrual bleeding. Most often it relates to menorrhagia (heavy bleeding) during your period. But it can also relate to:

- menstrual cycles that are shorter than twenty-four days
- menstrual cycles that are longer than thirty-eight days
- menstrual cycles that vary in length by more than seven days
- bleeding in between periods
- bleeding after sex
- bleeding after menopause

Why it happens: Various reasons. Fibroids, for example, can cause heavy periods that lead to you soaking through a tampon in just an hour. But so can a hormonal imbalance triggered by polycystic ovarian syndrome (PCOS) or a thyroid condition.

How to treat it: The first step is noticing that what's happening isn't normal. Track your symptoms and talk to your doctor about them so you can name your problem and find a solution. Fibroids can be treated with surgery.

Amenorrhea

What it is: Not getting your period by age fifteen or missing at least three menstrual periods in a row when you're not pregnant or breastfeeding. This one drives my Coochie-Chondriacs crazy.

Why it happens: It can be as simple as being stressed out or as complicated as a structural abnormality in your uterus. Your birth control (some contraceptives, particularly long-acting reversible contraceptives) can eliminate your period, as can allergy medications, blood pressure drugs, antidepressants, and antipsychotics, among others.

How to treat it: Work with your doctor to figure out the source of your missing menstruation issue. Bloodwork and imaging tests (like ultrasound) will help him or her get to the bottom of the problem.

TOP QUESTIONS WOMEN ASK ME ABOUT THEIR PERIOD

"Is it really all right to have sex during my period?"

Let's be real: your partners know we have periods. Quite frankly, they wouldn't be here if their mother didn't get them. And you can remind them of that. But I do understand that the hesitation around this comes from some religious doctrines that prohibit sex during menstruation. I'm not going to come between you and God, but I will tell you what I believe as a medical doctor. And I want my Virgin Marys, Sanctified Snatches, and Coochie-Chondriacs to listen closely—because I know a lot of them are shaking their heads right now. Not only is it all right to have sex during your period, it's actually good for you. There's research showing that having an orgasm can be a great pain reliever for those of you who get cramps around that time of the month. Even if you're not looking for an au naturel Advil, if you feel like getting it on, go for it. A word of caution: if either of you have a sexually transmitted infection and are having unprotected sex, getting it on during your period puts you at an increased risk of getting or passing on that infection. It's more important that your partner wear a "hat" when it's raining red.

"If I skip a period, does that mean I'm unclean because my lining just stuck around?"

Definitely not—but a lot of my patients do believe this. No matter what the reason for skipping your period (you're on continuous birth control, you have PCOS, etc.), it doesn't make you "dirty." Remember, young girls, pregnant women, and menopausal women don't get periods either.

"Is there an odor associated with having a period?"

Other people might've told you no, but here's the real deal. Yes, there's a smell associated with having a period. But it shouldn't radiate through your clothes and won't embarrass you in public. I'm just saying that you or your partner (when you're intimate) may notice a slight metallic scent from the iron in your blood. It's nothing to worry about and it certainly shouldn't make you run out to buy a bunch of scented products or deodorizers. Remember, your Queen V doesn't like it when you present her with perfumes and douches.

"I had a dark period this month. Is that normal?"

Completely. Sometimes when you're painting the town red, it actually comes out brown. When that happens toward the beginning of your period, it could be leftover blood or tissue from your last period that never made it out. If it's in the middle of your period, it could be related to an iron-rich diet. If it's at the end of your period, it could just be that your flow slowed, giving it more time for oxidation (combining with oxygen), which can change its color from red to brown.

"I pass a lot of clots in my menstrual flow. Should I be worried?"

Fear not. Having dime- or nickel-size clots in your period blood is perfectly normal. Having clots that are quarter-size or larger, however, might be a sign of a problem like fibroids, polyps, or adenomyosis. They can also be painful since they clog up your vaginal canal, causing your uterus to have to spasm to get them out. So you'll want to talk to your OB-GYN about diagnosing and treating the problem.

"Why is my poop looser when I get my period?"

Coochie-Chondriacs spot this problem long before the rest of us. While we're not exactly sure why it happens, experts definitely point the finger at hormonal changes that occur during your cycle. Every woman reacts differently though. Some women experience bloating or constipation instead.

"Can you still get pregnant if you have your period?"

Absolutely. Don't doubt it for a second. Sperm can live in your uterus for up to five days. So if you're at the end of your period and quickly ovulate, those swimmers can still make contact.

RIDING THE COTTON PONY (AND OTHER WAYS TO CAPTURE YOUR FLOW)

Pads

It might as well say "start here" on the box, since this is what most of us begin with. Sticking these absorbent shields onto your underwear keeps you from having an accident but won't let you go swimming or do yoga without stressing out about half frog pose. They come in a variety of shapes, sizes, thicknesses, and materials. Some of my health-conscious patients prefer organic ones, although I'm not sure they're as absorbent as regular brands.

Tampons

Experts estimate that 70 to 80 percent of menstruating women use tampons, highly absorbent rolls of cotton that you insert into your vagina (using your finger or an applicator) and remove using a string. There's been some debate about the chemicals used to grow and bleach cotton, hence the rise in organic tampons. You can also find reusable tampon applicators, for those concerned about the accumulation of plastic on the planet.

Period Underwear

One of the newest players on the red field is period underwear, which looks just like regular underwear but has a highly absorbent, leak-resistant, and odor-trapping middle section that holds your flow. Virgin Marys and Sanctified Snatches who don't want to insert anything into them are likely to find this a convenient, environmentally friendly favorite. You do need to hand wash them after every use though.

Menstrual Cups

You insert these flexible silicone or rubber cups into your vaginal canal to collect the flow of blood. Yes, more so than a tampon, you have to be comfortable with your body to do this. And, yes, there's an art to removing them over a toilet so you don't make a mess. But you can wear them longer than a tampon and you'll save money (and the planet) since you can use the same one for up to four years. You can also find soft, disclike cups that are placed high in the vaginal canal. These ones aren't reusable, but they do last longer than tampons and you can have sex while they're in.

Free Bleeding

In case you missed it, some women are just letting it flow without pads, tampons, or anything to catch their blood. Though I certainly believe in personal freedom to do what you want with your body, when your rights start to spill onto other people's, that's a bit too much. How would you feel if another woman was free bleeding all over your new car seat or the last person who sat in your movie theater seat was letting it flow? Plus, we do know that infections can spread through blood, so you could be creating a health risk for others—and they could be doing the same to you.

SEX ON THE RED SEA: HOW TO GET IT ON WHEN YOU'RE ON YOUR PERIOD

Once you've decided it's perfectly fine (in fact, enjoyable) to have period sex, let's talk about how to avoid spot cleaning your sheets in the morning. First stop: the shower. Getting some in the shower completely eliminates any concerns you might have about cleanliness. Plus, your flow acts like added lubrication and it all goes down the drain for easy tidying up after the last ooh-ooh-ooh. You just have to be careful. It's slippery in there.

If you'd prefer to be between the sheets, consider wearing a diaphragm (which you need to be fitted for) or a soft menstrual disc (available in drugstores), which will contain your blood flow and, unlike a tampon, allow you to still have sex.

Finally, if you're free-flowing, be sure to put a dark-colored towel underneath you and perhaps have a washcloth near the bed to wipe off with after climax. They're much easier to clean than your mattress or sheets. But you're not going to bleed *that much* anyway, so don't stress about it!

WHAT HAPPENS WHEN YOU FORGET A TAMPON INSIDE YOU

It rarely occurs to the same person twice. (Once you've been down this road, you usually learn your lesson.) But don't be surprised if happens to you at some point. The drama of the forgotten tampon is a story many women have lived out. It could be because it was the end of your period and you completely forgot you had one in there. Or perhaps you forgot it was in there, had sex, and it got pushed so far you didn't see the string at all.

Regardless of the how, most women come into my office genuinely confused. "I don't know what's wrong," they tell me. What they do know is they've noticed a foul-smelling discharge. I'm not going to lie to you all: it usually smells bad. Really bad. Like, so bad I shut down the exam room on that day. Like, "Did someone die in here?" bad. That combination of blood, semen, and regular discharge mixed into a slowly decaying piece of cotton smells like someone has just died. It's no fun for you or for me—but it's critical that you come in for a visit. I can help you remove it and also check you for toxic shock syndrome (TSS). It's a serious, life-threatening condition caused by a proliferation of bacteria from using superabsorbent tampons or leaving a tampon in for too long.

Ready for a big surprise? This is the one and only time I'll tell a woman to douche. Your vaginal flora has already been disrupted and the bacteria has already traveled everywhere it can. Douching will help get rid of the smell and clear out a pretty traumatized vaginal canal.

WHEN WILL IT BE OVER? MANAGING MENOPAUSE

Last winter, I had a fifty-four-year-old Mary Jane patient who nearly broke down into tears during our appointment. She was terrified that she had early onset Alzheimer's. "I've been crying myself to sleep every night," she admitted with her shoulders slumped and eyes down. "I even have trouble remembering the names of my kids. I have to think for at least five seconds before it comes to me and I can call them."

My heart went out to her until I started asking her about her other symptoms. Turns out she was having night sweats, putting on a few pounds around her waist, and her libido was completely out the window. "Your problem isn't Alzheimer's," I reassured her. "It's brain fog. MJ, you're in menopause."

You know all the crazy stuff your body did in puberty? Well, it's déjà vu when your body goes into perimenopause (as your ovaries begin to shut down) and then menopause (once they're done). I call that transition "mature puberty." Menopause usually kicks in at an average age of fifty-one—plus or minus a few years. But to officially be in menopause, you need to have gone one year without a period. That's twelve consecutive months.

If you haven't, you're in perimenopause. That can last anywhere from a few months to four years.

In both perimenopause and menopause, your period starts playing hide-and-seek. (Remember that oldie but goodie from puberty? Or maybe you don't because this transition brings with it a bit of brain fog.) Instead of boldly making its first appearance, your pubic hair starts doing a slow fade to gray. And your hormones? They're all over the place. Welcome to hot flashes, mood swings, and night sweats.

On the one hand. you're probably excited that soon you'll never have to throw down cash for tampons or insert a menstrual cup ever again. On the other hand, you might be frustrated because your Juicy Lucy is gone. The drop in estrogen gives your Queen V less lubrication (nothing a little hormone therapy or vaginal rejuvenation can't help with).

We're not exactly sure what triggers the start of menopause, but we do know that it's related to a few factors, such as:

- your genetics (when did it happen for your mom?)
- your diet (eating a lot of refined carbs can bring it on early, while consumption of omega-3 fatty acids can delay it)
- your lifestyle habits (research shows smoking can hasten it, but a tea-drinking habit can delay it)
- your medical procedures (cancer treatments, like surgical removal of your ovaries, chemotherapy, and radiation can induce menopause)

The number one question most women have for me around menopause is: "When will it be over?" They're wondering when they can stop carrying around a personal fan or waking up in wet sheets. When will their hormones ease the heck up so they can coast through the rest of their life being "postmenopausal"? The transition tends to last about seven years. But instead of rushing to the finish line—which is different for everyone—I try to get women to redefine the not-always-a-laugh-a-minute female journey. This transition is a milestone to be celebrated—not a dreaded period to be frowned upon.

I once read that this transition is a moment to reestablish your principles, your priorities, and your passions. Knowing that the baby-making is behind you, I believe this is a moment when you can fully focus on self-confidence, self-awareness, and, most important, self-care. Ask yourself what that means to you, how you want to live out the next half of your life, and when you're going to start making changes of your own. I have a three-part plan for doing all this.

It's time to make over your mind-set. I don't want you to simply accept the fact that you're never going to be thirty again. I want you to embrace it. Instead of looking behind you—you're not going that way!—look to what's ahead of you. I hear so many women in my office say, "Ugh, I'm fifty-five." How about swapping those three depressing words for three uplifting ones: "I. Am. Alive!" Do you know how many breast cancer patients I've watched pass away who didn't make it to fifty-five? Women who were fighting to make it to menopause and would've loved to be able to say, "I. Am. Alive!"? Cherish the gift you've been given.

You can't anti-age, but you can manage age. I'm claiming 120 years. That's right, I plan on living that long. But I don't want to look like 120 when I get there. Yes, we're all going to age, but we can age gracefully. Your body has been programmed by God to do certain things—and He's also given us technology to manage aging. Maybe that means a little filler in your hands to make them look like they belong to a thirty-year-old. Perhaps it's time to consider bioidentical hormone pellets to help you beat belly fat and get your sexy back. Maybe that means getting information about that knee replacement surgery so you can place first in your age group for a marathon thanks to your new titanium joint. Or perhaps this is about focusing more on diet so you can beat an increased heart disease risk that comes with being postmenopausal. Whatever you need, take this new moment for self-care to talk to your doctor about what technology can make possible for you. This is a time to invest in yourself, your health, and your future.

Let's reassess your circle of friends. There's never been a better time to hang out with people a few decades younger than you. It's draining hanging out with older friends who keep saying, "Girl, I'm tired." It's rejuvenating hanging out with young friends who keep saying, "What are we going to do next?" All my BFFs are younger than me. That's how you stay young at heart, body, mind, and spirit.

POINT OF V: BE FRENEMIES WITH BENEFITS

In case you're wondering what ever happened to that soror and me, you should know that our rivalry is over, done with, and way in the past now. But that doesn't mean I regret it. We were both able to use that competitiveness to our advantage. It made us better students (there was no way I was letting her get an A if I didn't get one), sharper dressers (I had to stay on top of my fashion game every time I walked out my room), and highly desirable dating options (remember, we were trying to win that guy's heart). I think the frenemy relationship that women have with their periods can do the exact same thing. You can either let her win—passing up that pool party invitation and lying on the couch with a pint of ice cream—or you can let her get you to the next level. I'm hoping you level up. Keep track of her every move so you'll know how to outsmart her in any situation and even get the guy in the end. (I sure did.)

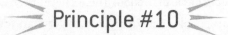

Principle #10

Know Your Breasts Like You Know Your Way Home

THE $450 SHIRT

Close your eyes and imagine getting a phone call from a doctor saying these four words: you have breast cancer. Just take a moment right now to stop and think about it. I'll wait.

So what happened? Did you feel fear swelling up in your chest? Did you sense some sadness strangling your spirit? Did your mind start racing to every scary possibility: hair loss, surgery, destruction of the life you've built for yourself, death? Did you feel numb, like all the feeling in your body had drifted away? Well, that was me. At 3:31 pm on February 23, 2004.

I knew I was supposed to wait patiently for my doctor to call me with the results of my recent biopsy. That's what any good patient should do. But as a physician, I knew exactly who in pathology to phone to get my left breast biopsy results as soon as they were in. And I was in Grind Mode. I wanted to check one more thing off my to-do list for the day— and I was sure he was going to say my results were negative. He had to say negative. I was in good health. I didn't smoke. I didn't drink alcohol. I had no family history of breast cancer. And I exercised often. My only risk factors for the disease were being female and not getting pregnant before the age of thirty. But I was hoping to get pregnant soon. Yes, I was certainly more than a few years late, but better late than never.

I made the call. They said they'd get back to me by lunch. But when

I hadn't heard anything by 3:30 pm, I dialed them up again—this time using my doctor status. I was put on hold for what felt like forever . . . And then. Then came the words I never thought I'd hear. Then came the moment the pathologist said, "You have infiltrating lobular carcinoma." I could feel my legs buckle as the words washed over me. How could I have cancer in my left breast?

"They must be giving me a patient's results," I thought. "Don't they know I'm calling about *my* results? About Dr. Jacqueline Walters's results? There must be some mix-up." The first stage of grief is denial. You just don't believe what's happening to you.

I never, not for one minute, not for one millisecond, ever thought I could have cancer. I got annual clinical breast exams from my partners at my practice and I did self-exams every month. Who better to check my breasts than me? Someone who does it more than forty times a day? You would think I know what breast cancer feels like. I know what it looks like. And I knew the uphill battle I was headed into as I picked up the phone and called my husband and my parents to tell them what I'd just heard.

When a surgeon becomes a patient, they're sort of standing on both sides of the knife. On the one hand, I was wearing a white coat and knew all the needles that were about to be injected into me, the surgeries that were going to be performed on me, the exact medications I'd need to take, and all the excellent percentages when it came to chances of survival from my stage I invasive lobular carcinoma. But as a patient with a flimsy paper gown on, I let go of all that knowledge and became consumed by how scary and unfamiliar so much of this was. I'd bounce back and forth between panic and calm, between reading (and rereading) the latest treatments and reading (and rereading) healing scriptures. In one moment, I'd be reassuring myself that things were going to be fine and in the next my eyes spontaneously welled up so much I couldn't see through my tears to perform a routine procedure on a patient.

Those two parts of me were at war with each other—but they needed to be in a unified fight against the cancer. I was facing a lumpectomy to remove the tumor and some tissue around it but preserve my left breast. Then I'd have six months of chemotherapy and thirty-three rounds of radiation. That would destroy any cancer cells that might have been left behind and decrease the chances of the cancer coming back. I won that battle. But the war wasn't over yet.

Four years later, I got my husband, Curtis, to go to the mall with me. I wanted to show him an Anne Fontaine top that I loved. One part was a white collared shirt, the other a black sweater. It was classy but had the shoulders cut out to look a little sexy too. It also had a sky-high, $450 price tag. Curtis looked at me and said, "Why don't we just buy it?"

What? I thought: "Is this man having an affair or done some other criminal act?" "Why are you being so nice to me?" I asked him. "What's gotten into you? I know my doctor didn't call and tell you I have breast cancer again. Did she?"

His face just sank.

This time around, I had been smarter about test results. I had been getting mammograms and/or MRIs every six months after finishing my treatment. But instead of calling the pathologist directly from my job— and having to deal with potentially devastating results by myself while still at work—I told my doctor to call Curtis instead. Once I saw that look on his face, I went right back into denial. This couldn't be happening *again*. What kind of sick joke was being played on me? But no, it was true. This time I was diagnosed with mucinous breast cancer in my right breast. It's a rare type of invasive carcinoma that accounts for only 2 percent of breast cancers. Two percent.

Breast cancer had tried to kill me. Not once, but twice. "It's either them or me," I thought when I agreed to get a double mastectomy. As devastated as I was, I was able to see a glimmer of meaning in my misfortune. "God," I said, searching for purpose in my pain, "you must have something really big planned for me."

If you were wondering why I'm taking a whole chapter to tell you about your breasts in a book that I promised would be all about your Queen V, this is your answer. That glimmer. That meaning. I share my story here, on stages across the country, and on television to make sure women realize that we're all at risk. One in eight women will be diagnosed with breast cancer in their lifetime. And if it could happen to a physician who believed herself to be healthy, then breast cancer can happen to you too. That's why it's so important to make sure that you know your breasts like you know the back of your hand. Like you know your way home. Like you know your BFF's deepest, darkest secrets. Breast cancer wasn't the end of my story. And this chapter is all about how to try to make sure that it isn't the premature end of yours either.

WHAT EXACTLY IS BREAST CANCER?

Your body is made up of about thirty trillion cells. Not million, not billion, but trillion—with a T. They've all got different jobs. Some are red blood cells carrying oxygen throughout your body. Others are fat cells, storing energy in your body. They can make it harder to squeeze into your favorite pair of jeans or a bit sexier when you slip into a bikini on vacation. Cells in your body die every day—and new ones are born every day in a healthy balance. When it comes to breast cancer, cells in your breast grow out of control. They form lumps and may also spread to other parts of your body (metastasize). While a woman is diagnosed with breast cancer every two minutes in the United States, you have to remember that this is a very treatable disease—especially when caught early.

A GUIDE TO GETTING TO KNOW YOUR GIRLS

If there's one message I want to get across to you from cover to cover, it's that you should advocate for your best sexual health when it comes to your lady parts—and I mean all your lady parts. But first we need to start with some basics.

First and foremost, let's define your breasts. Medically speaking, your breasts are fatty, fibrous, glandular tissue that sit atop your pectoral muscles and produce milk for babies when you give birth. Super-sexy medical jargon, right? Practically speaking, your breasts are like a celebrity power couple: attention-grabbing, envy-worthy, and at times an obsession. Breasts were all anyone could talk about when Janet Jackson had a "wardrobe malfunction" during the 2004 Super Bowl halftime show. They're one half of the duo that Kim Kardashian used to "break the internet." And they're the reason Sofia Vergara says she can't do push-ups. (Hey, there's always overhead presses.)

Besides caring for hungry babies and spooning with your partner, do they serve a purpose? Science hasn't quite figured that out yet. But what I can tell you is that like your vaginal flower, they come in different shapes and sizes.

You should also know that not every breast lump or bump is cancerous. Over 50 percent of women have fibrocystic breasts at some point in their life—a benign condition where your breast tissue feels lumpy or rope-like in texture and your chest may ache more right before your period. You might also feel benign cysts in your breast, which your doctor can aspirate.

Whether you're a Virgin Mary or a Notorious V.A.G., you need to do a better job supporting the girls that support you so you can avoid small problems (like awkward workouts) and overcome bigger ones (like cancer). Allow me to show you the way.

Step 1: See What You're Working With

Just like you did with your Queen V, give the Princess Bs a nice long look in the mirror. Breasts come in many sizes (AA to ZZZ), shapes (round or bell-shaped, relaxed or perky), positions (one may be perky, the other drooping), and symmetries (some are mirror images, others are asymmetrical). Not all of our headlights look the same. There are women with inverted nipples, and others have nipples that stick out or are flat. Notice what's different about yours. Is the left bigger? Or the right? Or do they appear exactly the same right down to every ridge of your nipple? It's important to know what your normal is so if that appearance ever changes, you'll notice. It's called breast "self-awareness," and many major health organizations are encouraging it.

While we're talking about looking out for your girls, let's talk about providing them with the right support. When was the last time you went to a lingerie department or store and got a bra fitting? That's what I thought: too long. In the US, 80 percent of women aren't even wearing the right bra size. (Think about that: Would you ever wear the wrong size panties? Or the wrong size shoes?) Here's the problem with that: when you're not wearing the right size undergarment, your girls aren't getting the TLC they need. It's not just that bra bulge and overflowing cups don't look cute. (Come on now, you know your clothes just don't look right when you're wearing the wrong bra. It's right up there with visible panty lines—worse, in my book—when it comes to fashion don'ts.) Wearing the wrong size bra can also lead to neck, shoulder, and back pain, and more. You're the chief health executive officer for these girls and you need to protect them. So your next move should be to get sized and then . . .

Step 2: Get in Touch with Yourself

While many doctors (including me) advocate doing monthly self-exams, many national organizations don't. Some research shows they're not helpful in finding cancers and may cause unnecessary testing. But I encourage women to keep feeling themselves up (and down and around). I've had two too many brushes with breast cancer, so I'm willing to do whatever it takes to protect my body—and yours.

Sure, your doctor may check them at least once a year. And your partner probably can't keep his or her hands off them either. But no one should know your breasts better than you do. You'll be the first to notice any dimpling, discoloration, discharge, thickening, lumps, or other changes to them so you can bring it to the attention of your doctor. Many of my patients who come to me with breast concerns are able to tell me "something's not right." Then they can take their hand and point me right to the area of concern. If you ever need to, I want you to be able to do the same with your doctor.

My recommendation to every woman in my office is to check their breasts the week after their period. Thanks to chemo and a drug called tamoxifen, I haven't had a period in years, so I choose to check my breasts on the twenty-seventh of each month. (That's the day I was born.) So that day every month I stand in the shower (and again in front of the mirror), lift one arm over my head, and feel away. If your breasts get sensitive during certain times of the month, don't use that as an excuse to skip your touch test. Pick another day when it won't hurt to do your monthly checks.

When you do a self-exam, don't be shy. Start by looking at your breasts in a mirror with your hands on your hips. Then give them a look holding your hands over your head. Next, keep your right hand raised while using the first few finger pads of your left hand to examine your breast from armpit to cleavage and from collarbone to abdomen. Some women like to make circles starting from the nipple and getting wider and wider. You could also go straight up or down like you do when shaving. Whatever method you choose, get in there with pressure like you would if you were kneading dough. Gently massage your breasts and see if any discharge comes from your nipples. Be sure to feel underneath your armpit to check your lymph nodes there too. Breast tissue juts underneath there a bit too, and cancer can sometimes start there. Once you're done massaging your right side, follow the exact same process to explore your left side, taking it from the west to the east.

You're not done yet! The last move is to lie down, place your left arm behind your head, and do the same technique to examine your breast with your right—just from a different position. Repeat that on the right side and then consider yourself checked.

Step 3: Watch for the Four Ps of Change

Breasts start forming when you're in the womb. That's right. Before you've let out your first cry for your mother's milk, your breasts are taking shape. They're on the move again when you hit the first P: puberty. This is the point in life where girls start to become sexually mature. Developing breasts are usually the first sign of puberty, right along with sprouting pubic hair and getting your first period. It doesn't happen overnight. It's a gradual process that begins with your nipple protruding, your areola getting larger, and your breast tissue getting larger. While I don't want you to panic, it's important to know that lumps appear in women of all ages. If a lump is ever felt in a girl entering puberty, it should be examined by a doctor. Chances are it's benign—likely a fibroadenoma, one of the most common masses found in adolescents. They're part of the fibrocystic breast condition that I mentioned earlier and see all the time in women in their twenties and thirties.

The second P is your period. Fluctuating hormones as your body prepares your milk ducts for pregnancy can lead to changes in your breasts like swelling and soreness. You might also notice a change in the texture of your breasts. (That's yet another reason why you should wait until a few days after you're done with tampons and pads for the month to do your check.) Some women who struggle with breast changes right before their period have fibrocystic breasts. To help with any pain, I tell my patients to try taking evening primrose oil or 400 IU of vitamin E once a day.

Now, I do have some Coochie-Chondriac and Mary Jane patients who are on top of their breast changes all throughout the month—not just when PMS strikes. They notice even a slight difference. (Kind of like when you were a kid and your momma noticed that a cushion on the couch had been flipped—only to discover that it's because you spilled some fruit punch on it.) These patients will tell me, "Every time I get my period, I feel something here" or "When it's that time of the month, I'll see something there." If that sounds like you, be sure to make an appointment to meet with your doctor (at least once) while you're menstruating so you can point out the change and have it checked.

The third P is pregnancy. Just like with puberty, changes in your breasts are one of the early signs that you're going to have a baby. Once again, those changes are thanks to your hormonal fluctuations. Your body is getting your breasts ready to become milk production factories, which can result in swelling, soreness, and tingling. If you feel a lump during pregnancy—which is not uncommon, by the way—don't assume that it's a blocked milk duct or some other change you can ignore. Talk to your doctor. I usually schedule my patients for a breast ultrasound after they've had a week to use warm compresses on the lump. Occasionally breast cancer is diagnosed in someone who is pregnant. But I don't want you to panic. Less than 5 percent of breast cancers are diagnosed in women under the age of forty. The most important thing is to pay attention to the changes in your body so we can keep mother and baby safe.

The last P is perimenopause and menopause. Hormones are at it again—this time with a drop in estrogen. In this stage, you'll lose some of the elasticity and fatty tissue in your breasts. This is the time in which your risk for breast cancer goes up. When you do your monthly checks, you'll notice that you feel a more grainy, lumpy, and irregular texture. If you're concerned about something you find, make an appointment with your doctor. I always say it's easier to cancel an appointment than to get one on the books. (Just make sure you call to cancel.) The median age for breast cancer diagnosis is sixty-two, so this is the time when you should be most on the lookout.

Step 4: Know Your History

It's time for you to have a slightly awkward conversation with your mother, your grandmother, and anyone who can give you a good answer about family health history. You need to know if anyone in your circle ever had breast, ovarian, and/or prostate cancer. Because women (especially in old school African American families) sometimes try to keep this a secret and the knowledge may not have been passed down, you may have to try asking the question in different ways. Ask: "Did anyone ever have any problems with their breasts?" Or, "Did anyone ever have breast surgery?" Take note of whatever you find out and report it back to your doctor when he or she asks about family history.

If you're adopted or your close family members are no longer living, that's another conversation to have with your MD. You can say, "Because I don't know my family history and we're learning a lot about the genetics of cancer, I want to know if I'm at increased risk. Are there any tests I can take for this?" Then see what he or she recommends.

Step 5: Show Up for Your Essential Exams

Most medical organizations don't recommend clinical breast exams—not even if you're at an increased risk of breast cancer. But you'll find that a lot of gynecologists still do them at your annual checkups. Some doctors may speed through them, but I take my time and really get in there because of my past experience. While I'm doing it, I think, "I hope this patient understands my passion for thorough examinations!" I'm just looking out for your best health.

Recommendations for mammograms, breast ultrasounds, and MRIs are a lot like little kids at a playground—they're really hard to keep up with, but it's so necessary that you do! Every organization's guidelines seem to be a little bit different. One organization says start at this age. Another says start later. The United States Preventive Task Force, which influences health insurance coverage, currently recommends getting mammograms every other year starting at age fifty, assuming you don't have a family history of the disease. But if I had followed those guidelines, I could have been in trouble. I didn't have a family history, but the first time I was diagnosed, I was just forty years old. And the second time I was forty-four, neither of which is at their recommended age.

My best advice is to develop a plan with your doctor that you both feel comfortable with, that won't have you stressed over unnecessary testing, and that won't have you paying out of pocket for tests (even though early detection would be a pretty good return on investment). In my practice, I order baseline mammograms for women at thirty-five. I've spoken with colleagues who are breast surgeons and they're very supportive of this practice that gives us an early image to compare with any future changes in your breasts.

Step 6: Check Your Genes

Genetics and family history account for only about 15 percent of breast cancer diagnoses. Allow me to do some important math on this for you.

That means that 85 percent of breast cancer diagnoses, the vast majority, have nothing to do with mutated genes (like BRCA1 or BRCA2) or your relatives (which include your dad, by the way). But it's easy enough to find out if your genetic pool puts you at increased risk for the disease. So I tell my people, if they qualify for genetic testing (or are willing to pay for it) and their doctor recommends it, get it. Early detection is your best protection. And it doesn't get any earlier than looking into your body's tiniest building blocks.

It would be wonderful if everyone could just get tested and be reassured. But it doesn't work that way. There's a long list of potential reasons you would be advised to go through the process and have your insurance company pay for it. They include everything from having a personal history of breast cancer before fifty to having a family history of ovarian cancer, pancreatic cancer, male breast cancer, or aggressive or metastatic prostate cancer. There are direct-to-consumer genetic test kits (like 23andMe) that promise to offer you some information for a great price, but the results are limited, so you might get a false sense of reassurance if you test negative. Trust me, this is truly a journey that you want to take with your doctor—not solo.

YOUR WHOLE-BODY APPROACH TO FIGHTING BREAST CANCER

If you've been diagnosed with breast cancer, it's time to accept your new norm. It won't be easy, but it's absolutely essential. One thing that helped me was getting one big, ugly, nasty cry out. Just letting myself scream, yell, and cuss. Do whatever you need to do to release the anger, fear, and frustration you're feeling. You're going through something traumatic, and on this journey it's too hard to fight with tears in your eyes.

After you've wiped them away, it's time to come up with a whole-body strategy for getting through the months ahead of you. It's not just about focusing on what's happening in your breasts, it's about taking control of how you move, what you put in your mouth, what you think, and more.

So when women ask me for advice about fighting breast cancer and coming out a winner on the other side, I offer a head-to-toe approach that starts with their mind-set.

Your Head: Know What You're Up Against

Once your doctor does a biopsy, they should be able to tell you a few key pieces of information that will determine your treatment plan.

- **Type.** Contrary to what a lot of people believe, there isn't just one type of breast cancer. There are many different types. The type of breast cancer you have is directly related to the cells in your breast that are affected. Some start in the milk ducts or milk-producing glands of your breast. In ductal carcinoma in situ (DCIS), which impacts one in five women newly diagnosed with breast cancer, the cells of your milk ducts are cancerous, but the disease hasn't spread beyond their walls. It's actually considered a "pre-cancer," and some women opt to take a wait-and-see approach for treatment. Other types of breast cancer start in the muscle, fat, or connective tissue of your breast. Phyllodes tumors, for example, develop in the connective tissue and are usually benign.
- **Stage.** The stage of your breast cancer explains how far the cells have spread and also what your chances of survival are. A stage 0 cancer, like DCIS, is the earliest stage. Stage IV is the most advanced stage of the disease, where it has spread to other parts of your body like your bones, lungs, liver, or brain. It's worth noting that the five-year relative survival rate for women fifteen to forty-nine with metastatic breast cancer has doubled in past years. It's not a death sentence. It turns cancer into a chronic illness like diabetes or hypertension.
- **Hormone receptor status.** The answer to this question determines whether hormone treatments will be helpful in treating your disease. Your cancer is considered hormone receptor positive

if the cells biopsied contain proteins (hormone receptors) that grow when exposed to hormones (estrogen or progesterone). Your cancer is considered hormone receptor negative if they don't. You'll hear the phrases ER+ (estrogen receptor-positive) or PR- (progesterone receptor-negative). You should also be tested to determine your HER2 status (human epidermal growth factor receptor 2). This protein on the surface of some breast cancer cells impacts cell growth as well.

Before you make any permanent decisions about your treatment plan, take time to make sure you understand the situation you're in. You're about to be hit with a lot of medical jargon and it's important that you understand what it all means for you.

You've got to have a rock-solid relationship with your doctor as they talk you through your diagnosis and your treatment plan. If you don't understand something that she's saying, be honest. Asking questions actually builds trust between the two of you—it doesn't tear it down. I view answering questions as a key part of my job. You didn't spend seven years getting a medical degree. I did. So it's my responsibility to help you understand what's happening in your body.

I always ask my patients if they're clear on what I've explained to them and if they have any more questions before I leave the exam room. If your doctor isn't comfortable answering your questions or can't explain things in a way that you understand, it's time to move on to another doctor. If I can't figure something out, I'll find someone else who can. I surround myself with smart people—and you should too.

One more thing: while you may want to move on if you can't get to a place where you understand your doctor, you don't have to leave if you disagree with your doctor. I've had patients challenge me on getting a particular test or going through a particular procedure. That's okay. I'm still here to help them and I'm still on their team. At the end of the day, it's your body and you get to decide how to care for it. And it's your money, so if you choose a test that isn't covered by your plan, you'll have to pay for it.

Your Mouth: Preach Positivity

I need you to stay positive. Even though what's happening to you is the very definition of unfair, even though you're in a lot of emotional and maybe physical pain, and even though you might be angrier than you have ever been in your life, you've got to steer clear of the negative. I say this for science's sake. Your immune system's response is better when you're positive. People are drawn to you when you're positive. (I'm thinking of those helpful nurses you'll be needing and the busy doctors you'll be calling at odd hours.)

Find a way to allow nothing but positive statements to come out of your mouth. As I was fighting breast cancer, you couldn't get me to own the disease. I never said, "my breast cancer." I'd say "the breast cancer diagnosis." I never said "I'm sick." I told people "I'm going through healing." I read every scripture about healing there is in the Bible. I'd put on headphones at night and listen to positive motivation CDs as I slept.

Words have power, but you have to find the ones that work for you and your situation. Maybe when you wake up in the morning, remind yourself, "I am becoming stronger every single day." When you look in the mirror in the bathroom, tell yourself, "I am a fighter!" When you're sitting in a waiting room at your doctor's office, keep thinking to yourself, "I will be cancer-free."

Your Eyes: Keep Looking Beautiful

We all know that if you look good, you feel good. That's why I started the 50 Shades of Pink breast cancer foundation. We're not only helping men and women diagnosed with breast cancer navigate the healthcare system. We're supporting their inner beauty and their outer beauty as well. We want them to get through the process of fighting breast cancer *looking* unscathed. That's something different for everyone. It might mean shaving your head and rocking a baldie. It could be picking out a bright pink wig. It might be that you never leave the house without your favorite shade of lipstick on. Or that you always step out in a pair of heels that make you feel sexy and confident. Find what reminds you of the beautiful woman you are and flaunt it as much as you can.

Your Heart: Let People Help You

So often we as women feel like we have to be in control of everything. But I'm giving you permission to not have it all together during moments of this fight. Hold on, scratch that. I'm telling you to expect to have periods of time when you feel like you don't have it all together. You can't do it all. But you can keep putting one foot in front of the other and let your support system lighten your load while you're moving forward.

How? Bring your spouse, your sister, or a close friend with you to your appointments to make sure you're clear on everything the doctor is telling you. (You might be overwhelmed and not thinking straight.) Ask a friend to pick up groceries for you if you just can't pull it together to make it out of the house today. My best friends were a big part of the support group I created for myself. They went to appointments with me for emotional support, consoled me when I cried uncontrollably, and laughed with me when I needed cheering up. Yes, even doctors go through all the feelings!

Only you know who'll get invited into your inner circle for support, but let me say this: you know who the warriors are in your family and you need to link arms with them. I love my momma, but when she heard I had breast cancer the first time, she was catatonic on her couch for hours. I couldn't put the weight of my treatments on her. I didn't tell her when I was going through chemotherapy. You'll need to spend some time thinking about who you can lean on when you're in the trenches and then speak up. Call them when you're scared and tell them, "I just need you to listen to what's going on." Text them and ask them if they can watch your kids for a few hours because you need a break. Email them and see if they can come to an appointment with you and take notes so you don't miss anything. I'm more likely to help a friend—and go out of my way to do so—when she tells me what's going on. But if I don't know, what can I do?

I do believe that everyone should consider a therapist during a traumatic time in their life. I encourage you to not just talk but also listen. Get out what you need to say but also spend time considering the questions your therapist asks you. Take action on the coping mechanisms he or she offers. It may be more convenient or affordable for you to go to an organized support group. I know they are incredibly powerful experiences for a lot of people, but I personally felt like I was being pounded with negativity at the first one I went to. To this day, I remember the voice of one man in my group telling us all in a thick Southern accent that his cancer came back. That group wasn't for me. If you realize that your group isn't building you up—instead it's breaking you down—find another one.

Your Hands: Get a Journal. Stat.

I tell everyone to purchase a journal when they're first diagnosed. (It's part of the 50 Shades of Pink breast cancer support baskets we create.) Getting a journal was one of the first things I did when I was diagnosed. Yes, you can use it to write down your feelings. If you can't bring yourself to scream aloud, you can do it in all caps and giant letters across the entire page. If there are fears that you're afraid to say to someone else, you can write them down on the pages of your book. But what I used my journal most of the time for was information-gathering. I'd ask a friend, "Who did your girlfriend go to for a second opinion?" and then add that name to a growing list of the names of recommended doctors in my book. I'd ask someone in a support group, "What hospital are you going to?" And then jot that down. I'd keep track of appointment dates, times, and locations. I could also write down notes from research on breast cancer I had read. It was helpful to have one convenient place to capture all my thoughts, ideas, and, most importantly, my plans of action.

Your Hips: Keep Your Money Straight

I'm talking about the cash in your pocket. You didn't see that one coming, did you? Here's the problem. Most people get diagnosed and only focus on one thing: not dying. But the world keeps spinning even when something terrible has happened to you. You have to make sure that you keep money coming in. Your boss may be angry if she notices you're calling in sick all the time—unless you've sat down and had a conversation with her about your illness. I've seen women get fired because they waited too long to tell their employer why their productivity was down and they were showing up less often. Make sure to keep your job in the loop so they don't assume you're at interviews when you're really getting chemo. Instead of explaining past behavior, give them a heads-up as to what to expect.

You also have to make sure that money keeps going out. Georgia Power is going to cut off your lights unless you make your way through the pile of bills on your kitchen counter—even when you're feeling depressed. Think about automatic bill payment or have a friend come over and help you get through the stack of mail.

"SO WHAT HAVE YOU BEEN EATING?"

I've had patients push back their appointments by a month or two so they could lose a few more pounds before coming to see me. It's not the scale they're afraid of. It's me bringing up what's on the scale that they fear. Most people know how passionate I am about healthy living.

After my battles with breast cancer, I knew I wanted to be as healthy as possible. Obesity is directly linked to breast cancer: being overweight or obese after menopause increases your risk of the disease because it increases your estrogen levels. Not to mention that excess body weight ups your risk of a host of other illnesses like diabetes, hypertension, and more. So I made diet and exercise changes and tried to bring others along with me by starting a Fit Is The New It initiative at my practice. (They call me Dr. FITNI.) They see me sticking my fork in salads on *Married to Medicine*. They watch me doing burpees, lat pulldowns, and leg presses with my trainer of fifteen years on my Instagram feed. Twice a week, I wake up at five a.m. (if I've had the luxury of sleep) and get to the gym in my camouflage spandex. No excuses. That's what it takes to fight obesity, stay strong, and level up.

Most physicians stay away from talking about weight because it's a sensitive topic. But I don't think I'm doing my job if I'm not open, honest, and still gentle with you about all aspects of your health. It would be like only giving you half an exam but charging you the full price. I'd be stealing your money by allowing you to walk out of my office thinking that your body weight is fine if I've crunched the numbers and I know it's not. So I've become the Ideal Body Weight Police—but I assure you I patrol with courtesy, professionalism, and respect. I'm here to protect, serve, and do no harm.

Now there's a nice little bonus when it comes to laying down the law about my patients' weight. Slimming down can change your VP. When you lose a significant amount of weight, the fat above your pubic area (the mons pubis) decreases. You could look better in tight dresses without that bulge right there. People start to notice. And you start to feel hotter. I've seen many women who were overweight Mary Janes at their last annual appointment but came to me the next year at their ideal body weight feeling like a Notorious V.A.G. Or they were a worried and obese Coochie-Chondriac who came back happier and lighter as a Mary Jane. Is eating healthy and exercising easy? No. Is it worth it? Absolutely.

I don't have a magic formula for you to follow to slim down. I'm not going to preach the virtues of intermittent fasting or tell you to join Cross-Fit. But there are a few golden fitness rules I recommend to everyone that can help them stay in shape.

Golden Rule #1: Eat Live

If it comes in a bag or a box, bye-bye! (Well, unless they're frozen fruits and veggies in a bag.) Here's the issue: processed foods are a big part of what's getting Americans in trouble with extra pounds. When you eat live, you avoid them. Eating live means that if you don't kill it (like chicken) or grow it (like broccoli), you limit it. Notice I didn't say avoid it. I'm not that harsh. But I believe about 80 percent of weight loss is tied to your diet. If you can control that, more than half the battle is won.

Golden Rule #2: Avoid Fruit Juices and Soda

When you separate fruit from its fiber, you're basically just drinking sugar. Which is excess calories. Which can lead right back to weight gain. Reach for water instead.

Golden Rule #3: Follow the 3 Bs of Cooking

Bake, boil, and broil. With healthy ingredients. If you start to add butter and cream to your dishes, that only ups the fat content. Now I'll be honest, I can't eat a black bean burger without a little bit of mayo. But it's about moderation. I don't bite into one every week. More like once a month.

Golden Rule #4: Keep Moving

Find workouts you love (dancing, hopping on the elliptical trainer, going hiking with your girls) and make them a habit most days of the week. If you asked me to get on a stationary bike, I'd roll my eyes. But I love walking outside to get my steps in. You can't beat the mood-boosting endorphin rush that comes from working out—even on days you think you're too tired. Plus you'll keep being able to fit into your little black dress.

THE TRUTH ABOUT *NOT* GETTING TESTED

While writing this book, I asked my Instagram followers for the reasons why they don't get tested for breast cancer. I've officially heard every excuse in the book—and I have an answer for them all. Are you ready for some tough love? Because that's what I'm about to dish out to you ladies.

Patients say: Breast cancer treatment kills more than it saves.
I say: What now? Where in the world did you hear that?

Actually, I have an idea. Many women get their health information from a group of people I call the "street committee." They believe the people around them (friends, neighbors, coworkers) have their best interest at heart more than any doctor would. There's also some distrust of doctors in certain communities. There's an expectation that doctors should be perfect—like God. But that just isn't the case. So when mistakes happen, that bond gets broken. So let me tell you the research-based facts. If you look at any study, far more people die from lack of treatment than would ever die from treatment. In the past three decades, as many as 614,000 deaths from breast cancer have been *averted* thanks to mammography and advances in treatment.

Patients say: My work situation is complicated and I don't have
   health insurance.
I say: There are tons of workarounds.
So many organizations offer reduced-cost or free mammograms all across the country. You can search for one on the internet or call your local hospital and inquire.

Patients say: Genetic testing is definitely too expensive.
I say: Our greatest wealth is our health.
The problem is most people don't invest in their health. They'd rather throw down money for a house, a car, fancy shoes, or gorgeous nails. All those things can disappear and come back to you. But your health? That's one thing you may not be able to get back if it's taken from you. I can't tell you how to spend your money, but I can encourage you to think long and hard about what's most important to you in life.

Patients say: I don't want to know if I have breast cancer.
I say: Do you want to know what your son looks like on his wedding day? Do you want to know what it would be like to go on
   a mother-daughter trip with your momma next year?
I have a Mary Jane patient who found a lump while she was breast-feeding her second child. She came into my office that same day and said,

"What do I need to do? Because I want to be around for my two kids and my husband, so what's the plan?" I'm not saying it's easy. The meds wore the Mary Jane out when she was already being run ragged as a mom. She also gained a fair amount of weight from the drugs that she needed to take. But she took charge and she's one year cancer-free now. I think of her when people say, "I don't want to know." Really, it's a bit selfish. They're only thinking of themselves. You're not just making a decision for yourself when you say, "I don't want to know." You're making a decision that will impact your family, your friends, your employer, and all the people who love and depend on you.

Patients say: I don't have time!

I say: You're costing yourself time.

You might be subtracting precious days, weeks, months, or years from your life by not getting tested. You can do a self-exam in the shower or during the commercial breaks of your favorite show. In the hour that you'd spend at a doctor's appointment getting screened, you could skip seeing one terrible movie every year or one trip to a department store.

Patients say: I won't feel empowered by the knowledge. I'll feel
       weakened or weighed down by worry.

I say: Worrying is a negative meditation.

You're dwelling on a potentially bad outcome when you really don't know what your results will be. Instead of putting all your attention on the negative, switch your thoughts and your vision to the positive. One in eight women will get breast cancer in their lifetime. That means seven out of eight won't. Tell yourself, "I'm empowered enough to know I have choices." Admit, "I don't want to get breast cancer, but if I do, I'm going to fight it and win." I did this during my treatment and I still do it today. When I'm pulling together a fundraiser for my 50 Shades of Pink Foundation, I don't worry about how many tickets we'll sell. I envision a sold-out gala and then I turn my attention to more promotion.

Patients say: Mammograms hurt.

I say: You're right. I'm afraid they do hurt. But not more than
    cancer.

A ten-minute mammogram is uncomfortable. Later-stage breast cancer
often involves chemotherapy treatments, radiation treatments, and surgery. That's a whole lot more painful. And you may be able to avoid some
of that pain with an earlier diagnosis.

Patients say: I have fibrocystic breasts, so going through all that
    testing gets frustrating.

I say: Flip those feelings.

Instead of being frustrated, you should be celebrating every time your
doctor reassures you that you've got a clean bill of health or you do a self-
check and don't find anything. Frustrating is missing a lump because you
didn't get a mammogram last year. Getting a green light after showing up
is a reason to rejoice.

Patients say: I'm too terrified to get tested.

I say: Don't run scared. Let's catch this disease before it catches
    you.

If you're dragging your heels over scheduling a mammogram, remember that the sooner you find cancer, the more options you'll have. And that
a negative test result could inspire you. You can decide to change your
lifestyle by eating healthier foods and exercising more. Don't cross your
arms and refuse to take action. Use all the tools you've been given to make
the best of whatever health situation you find yourself in.

THE SPECIALIST'S CORNER: BREAST CANCER

When a doctor reveals the name of the person she goes to with her own
health problems, you should listen up. It's a pretty big deal—and it's exactly
what I'm about to do here. After I was diagnosed with breast cancer, one

name rose to the top of the list of people I was willing to trust with my life: Jennifer L. Amerson, MD. As a surgeon at Breast Cancer Specialists in Atlanta with more than twenty years of experience in the field, she was my go-to. Here's our "V" Q&A on overcoming our fears around breast cancer, finding the best surgeon possible, and what you must know about the latest advances in the field.

Dr. Jackie: There's so much fear and uncertainty around getting diagnosed with breast cancer and choosing the right treatment. What's your best advice for women on dealing with that?

> **Dr. Amerson:** Breathe! This is one situation where time is not of the essence. Breast cancers have generally been there at least four years before becoming apparent on imaging. It is more important to take your time to gather all the necessary information you need to make the right decision rather than rush into surgery. It's also important to realize that the five-year survival rate for breast cancer is very high at 90 percent. The average woman's chances are very good.

Dr. Jackie: What should a patient be looking for when you're searching for a good breast cancer specialist?

> **Dr. Amerson:** Find someone who has a special interest in breasts and does more than 50 percent of their surgeries in that area. The surgeon should be comfortable reading breast imaging. Most important, you should be comfortable with the surgeon.

Dr. Jackie: Can you give women some questions they should ask the diagnosing doctor when they're told they have breast cancer?

> **Dr. Amerson:** I would want them to go into depth with the pathology. Be able to review the films. Ask them, "What are my surgical options? Lumpectomy, mastectomy, oncoplastic surgery—which

is breast reconstruction?" Don't be afraid to speak up. If you don't understand a concept, ask the surgeon to go over it again. There are no dumb questions. It is important for you to be on board and know all the options to make good decisions.

Dr. Jackie: I think a lot of women assume that breast cancer means you'll need chemotherapy, but that's not the case, right?

Dr. Amerson: True. The decision to recommend chemotherapy is dependent on characteristics of the cancer such as estrogen receptors and HER2 status. Size of the cancer does not determine the need for chemotherapy.

Dr. Jackie: How has breast cancer treatment evolved over the last five to ten years?

Dr. Amerson: A new tool for the oncologist is the Oncotype Dx score, which looks at the actual genetics of the cancer. The oncotype is the most important advancement over the past few years in the treatment of cancer. There are also so many new ways to treat breast cancer with newer drugs targeted specifically to the type of breast cancer the patient has.

POINT OF V: BOLDLY TAKE YOUR HEALTH INTO YOUR OWN HANDS

There's a difference between being an adult and being grown. Women who are adults have their age chronologically bestowed upon them. Women who are grown make responsible decisions regardless of age. They weigh the consequences, take action, and deal with the outcomes of their decisions. Part of being grown is holding your health in your own hands carefully—and not dropping it. I've had to do this twice in my life. I told you about the second time, when I thought, "God, you must have something big planned for me." I was right. That's when I started planning and I learned to use my power to empower others.

Since then, as I mentioned, I've created the 50 Shades of Pink Foundation for breast cancer warriors. I've boldly posed seminude—and got my friends to do it too—to raise money for breast cancer. And I've walked countless miles as a part of national fundraisers. My experience has made me a better doctor. I don't think there's ever an easy way to get bad news. But because I've survived breast cancer—twice—I can give bad news in a different way. I always start out by saying, "I don't have good news, *but* I've been there and I can certainly help you go down this path."

If you've been diagnosed, don't see it as a be-all and end-all. There are treatment options that improve the survival rate of breast cancer. Your diagnosis isn't the end of the road. It's the beginning of your journey. Know your treatment options. Find a support system. Don't go it alone. And get ready for battle.

If You Don't Control Your Fertility, It Will Control You

"WHICH CHILD IS YOURS?"

A year after getting married, I was ready to be both a wife and a mother. I wanted a smart and adorable baby. A girl, if I'm being honest. One who didn't have to feel intimidated by her six-foot-nine father should she end up my height. I knew that in order to make the invisible visible, you have to set goals. My first goal was to make sure that I was healthy. So I got a mammogram—and that fateful breast biopsy I already told you about that detected the cancer.

Now, at the time of that mammogram, I was already at the end of an inevitable pregnancy loss. I was spotting way too much and was sure this was unlikely to be a healthy pregnancy. I was going to lose that baby. After all, I'm an OB-GYN. I could read the signs. I thought I'd just get my mammogram, be in the clear, and be ready to try again in the next months. But I was wrong. Then I made what I thought was an innocent phone call. And there I was: pregnant, spotting, slowly passing tissue that I knew was the little person whom I had already envisioned and started to prepare my life for, learning that I was losing a baby, and accepting that I had to fight breast cancer all at about the same heartbreaking, terrifying time.

Once I finished half a year of chemotherapy, six months of radiation, and two years on tamoxifen—which was supposed to be five years, but I stopped early—I got back to my goals. But after several months of trying and tracking my irregular (oftentimes absent) cycles, I saw a reproductive endocrinologist who gave it to me straight: "You're not going to get pregnant naturally," she said.

Even though I had stopped getting regular periods and my FSH and LH levels (key indicators of fertility) were way too high, I didn't want to believe her. I was going to be a mother. I had stacks of ovulation kits I knew would eventually prove my doctor wrong. Every month I was peeing on those sticks to figure out when I was ovulating. Then I'd run and tell Curtis, "I've got an egg! We need to be having sex now!" Then I'd wait to feel breast tenderness, nausea, cravings for pickles, or just see a plus sign on a pregnancy test. But nothing happened.

After months of that not working, I started taking Clomid, a fertility medication to help me ovulate and perhaps produce more than one egg. As a doctor, I knew all my body's signs were saying I was menopausal. But as a patient, I was in denial. This *was* going to happen for me. What I knew as a doctor (that this wasn't going to work) never once came into play because my innate desire to be a mother overtook the medical knowledge I had.

It was often downright depressing for me to go to work and hear that my patients got pregnant using the tips I'd shared with them. The advice went both ways. Anything they told me, or that I heard on the news or read on the side of a bus, I'd try. Acupuncture? Sure. Chinese herbal teas? Let's give them a try. Short of standing on my head, I did everything— and it was exhausting. Every month I felt like I was running a race, getting so close to the finish line . . . and then someone moved the line half a mile down the road. Again. And again.

In the midst of all this, I was also working really hard to stay healthy after my bout with breast cancer—and sometimes that worked against my baby dreams. I should've still been taking tamoxifen, but as I mentioned, I stopped against my doctor's recommendations so I could try to get pregnant. I started being what I call a fegetarian (fake vegetarian) to be super healthy (while still sneaking in some chicken here and there). But I might not have been getting enough of a balanced diet, and I knew I wasn't getting enough protein because my hair started falling out.

I wasn't in control of my fertility at all. It was in control of me. It was the boss of my emotional state. It could make me happy and optimistic because Curtis and I were trying, or it could make me depressed and angry because I got my period that month. Or I got no period and still had negative pregnancy tests. It was the boss of my body as I took these medications to stimulate my ovaries. And it was in control of my finances as I shelled out money for incredibly expensive fertility drugs, treatments, and appointments with specialists all over Atlanta who told me it just wasn't going to happen for me.

One of those appointments was with a reproductive endocrinologist a colleague told me about. "She's helped women just like you stimulate and retrieve eggs," she said. With the spark of hope that ignited inside me, I could barely wait to meet with her. But when Curtis and I sat down in her office, my excitement turned to sadness mixed with anger. Sure, she told me she had stimulated ovaries and gotten eggs in women over forty who had gone through chemo. But when I asked her how many of those women went on to have babies, she said zero. None. Not one. She may as well have just punched me in the stomach because that's how it felt. "What the hell am I here for?" I thought to myself. "I don't care about eggs. I care about babies!" I couldn't believe that I'd paid all this money for a consult just to hear her talk about her zero success rate.

After that, everything became a blur. I just wanted to get out of that office. The whole car ride home, Curtis and I sat in silence. I didn't say one word to him. I couldn't even look at him. I'd dragged him all the way to this office so we could hear what he already knew. That we should stop trying. But I still just couldn't believe it. So I turned to my mentor, another reproductive endocrinologist, for some uplifting advice. I thought she'd tell me what I wanted to hear and encourage me to keep trying. But, once again, I was wrong. "You need to stop," she said. "Think about adoption."

When everyone you know, love, and trust is telling you the exact same thing, it's hard to deny. I can't say that I completely gave up hope. I kept having sex hoping that maybe—just maybe—a miracle might happen. But the flame of my hope got a little dimmer and a little dimmer each day.

A few weeks later, I went to a high school basketball game that Curtis was coaching. As I sat in the bleachers listening to everyone cheering for their kids, the realization of where the past few years had left me hit me harder than I expected. I just wanted to cry. My brain started telling me a truth that I didn't want to hear. That I'd never be waking up early on weekends to get my kid to a basketball game. That I'd never be tossing a kid-size jersey into the washing machine. That I'd never get to sit here cheering for my child on the court with her sports-fanatic dad.

While my mind was racing through all the "nevers" I'd miss out on, the woman seated next to me at the game asked, "Which child is yours?"

I sat there for a moment, looking at the faces of all the kids scurrying up and down the court. Then I raised my hand and pointed to Curtis. "That one. The one who's coaching," I told her with a smile. Then I yelled really loud, "Good coaching!" so he could hear me.

WHAT IS INFERTILITY?

It can often be a dream deferred . . . and deferred . . . and deferred. It's getting your hopes up every month when you imagine you're creating a little baby—and then having those hopes dashed when you get your period a few weeks later. The medical definition of infertility is not being able to get pregnant after a year of trying. But if you're over thirty-five, you shouldn't wait twelve months to see a doctor. Women between thirty-five and thirty-nine should see a specialist after half a year of attempting to conceive, and women over forty should go to an MD within the first six months of failed attempts.

Just like thirteen, thirty-five can be an unlucky number—but when it comes to infertility. First, your fertility begins a steady decline. Your number of eggs goes down while your chances of the remaining eggs having chromosomal abnormalities that will prevent you from having a healthy pregnancy go up. Should you get pregnant (let's hear it for the boy! or girl!) you're considered to be of "advanced maternal age." That means there are some increased risks that come with your pregnancy. You're at higher risk of developing hypertension or diabetes during your pregnancy, you have a greater chance of needing a C-section, and there is a higher chance of your having a miscarriage. All this means you'll want a close relationship with a doctor you trust as you get older.

SEXUAL ANATOMY 103:
WHAT DRIVES YOUR FERTILITY

We covered all your external lady parts in Principle #1 and some spots along the vaginal canal in Principle #8. Now it's time to look at the key fertility players deep inside your Queen V. When it comes to getting pregnant, you should know the basics of these reproductive parts.

- **Hypothalamus and pituitary gland.** Babies on the brain is absolutely right. These neighboring sections of your brain work together to control menstruation and reproduction. They signal other parts of your body to produce hormones that mature and release eggs. When they stop doing so, for example, if you have hypothalamic amenorrhea, ovulation and menstruation cease, resulting in infertility.
- **Ovaries.** This is where the baby-making magic begins. Your left and right ovaries are each about the size of a walnut and they hold approximately 300 thousand eggs total by the time you hit puberty. Each month, an egg is released toward a fallopian tube, priming you to get pregnant. They also produce sex hormones, like estrogen, progesterone, testosterone, and others. When you enter menopause, that production goes haywire and then drops, causing hot flashes, decreased libido, brain fog, vaginal dryness, and other unpleasant side effects.
- **Fallopian tubes.** Each ovary has a long, narrow duct near it that your egg travels down to meet sperm each month. Similarly, sperm swim up into the fallopian tubes to meet the egg. Fertilization takes place inside the fallopian tube and then the fertilized egg continues down the tube into the uterus to implant. When ectopic pregnancies occur—a dangerous scenario in which implantation happens outside the uterus—they're usually within a fallopian tube and require medical or surgical intervention. When a woman has a tubal ligation, it severs or blocks these

four- to five-inch-long tubes so the egg and sperm never meet. Some experts believe that the most common form of ovarian cancer begins in the fallopian tubes. This theory may change the way we try to prevent the disease by allowing women at risk to remove their tubes but keep their ovaries (so they don't enter early menopause) and uterus (allowing them to still carry a baby).

- **Uterus.** When you're not pregnant, this cavity where babies grow is about the size of your fist. When a fertilized egg leaves the fallopian tube, it travels into your uterus and implants somewhere on its inner walls. Your baby spends the next forty weeks growing there, expanding your uterus to the size of a watermelon. After you give birth, it will take about six weeks for the uterus to return to its original size.

WHAT CAUSES INFERTILITY?

About one out of every ten women of childbearing age struggle with infertility—but the reasons are almost as numerous as the potential solutions. Sometimes, infertility is just a matter of time. While you might not care about how old you are, your biological clock is paying closer attention than a bouncer at a club. Women are born with about one million eggs, but as we get older that number declines. Sharply. In your lifetime you'll ovulate only 300 or 400 eggs. While that still may sound like a lot, know that there's a sharp downward turn in both number and quality of eggs when we hit our midthirties. Not only will you have fewer and fewer eggs to produce, but the ones left behind may not produce a healthy baby. As more women wait until later in life to get pregnant, it's important to remember those numbers. If you're in your forties, your chances of getting pregnant are less than ten percent.

Physical problems can be a cause of infertility. If your fallopian tubes are damaged, blocked, or missing, that can prevent your eggs from ever meeting up with sperm.

If you ovulate at irregular intervals because you're obese, underweight, under a tremendous amount of stress, or have a condition like PCOS, that can make it harder to conceive.

Genetic defects can also work against you, which makes it all the more important that you get tested to see if you're a carrier of any conditions like Turner syndrome, Fragile X syndrome, spinal muscular atrophy, muscular dystrophy, cystic fibrosis, or sickle cell anemia. Exposure to radiation or chemotherapy, which is what I went through with my cancer treatments, can diminish your ovarian reserve.

Even if you do conceive, a uterine abnormality that you were born with (like a septate uterus, which has a muscular band of tissue running down its middle) or that developed later in life (like fibroids and endometriosis) can make it harder for that embryo to implant itself in your uterus and a baby to grow there.

Most difficult of all, sometimes infertility has no explanation. Sometimes science can offer us a diagnosis with no cure. For example, we can diagnose subclinical endometritis but we can't cure it. Other times, science hasn't figured out what the problem is. I had a Sanctified Snatch who got pregnant eleven times—and lost the baby in the first trimester each and every time. I know that her heart broke with every single disappointment. It was painful treating her because there was almost nothing I could do—except support her if she wanted to try again.

Often, infertility has absolutely nothing to do with you at all. About 40 percent of infertility problems can be traced to your partner's sperm. It may be that he has a low sperm count or his swimmers have low motility. You and your partner will need to speak to a fertility specialist and a urologist to look into different options to solve the problem.

I'll never forget a Mary Jane patient of mine in her late thirties who spent ten traumatic years trying to get pregnant—but she and her husband were never successful. She was able to put on a brave face, surrounded by pregnant women in my waiting room. But once she got into my office she'd break down in tears. With infertility, doctors will run tests in an attempt to put together a puzzle that shows them what's holding you back from conceiving. But sometimes the pieces just don't fit together and they can't figure out what's gone wrong.

Eventually she not only had to give up on the dream of the family she wanted to create—but also the man she wanted to create it with. I can't say if infertility was the only reason, but the stress of it was probably one of the reasons she and her husband ended up getting divorced. So you can imagine my surprise when she showed up at her next appointment with me . . . almost fifty and pregnant. Thinking that she was infertile, she'd been messing around with a cute young lover—and she ended up getting a whole lot more than her groove back. The problem wasn't her eggs, it seemed. Maybe it was her husband's sperm.

HOW TO CONTROL YOUR FERTILITY THROUGH THE YEARS

When your fertility has taken charge of you—but you're desperate to take back control—it's almost like trying to stage a military coup against your Queen V and the fertile territory she reigns over. You're coming at her with all the money, science, and sheer hope you have either to get her to stop you from having a baby or to produce one.

But my hope for you is to never have the need to overthrow your Queen V or try to seize her power. Instead of a hostile takeover, I want you to be her closest confidant and trusted adviser. Someone who whispers brilliant plans into her ear about the perfect contraception, when would be ideal to get pregnant, and what the two of you will do about it together—not as part of an insurrection but as a unified force. Avoid turning your fertile kingdom into a battleground by maintaining constant control of your Queen V with these strategic moves:

√ Identify Your Fertility Status

Infertility can happen at absolutely any age. When my patients come to me after six months to a year of trying to get pregnant, depending on age, I'll check blood levels for hormones that impact pregnancy, we'll make sure that their fallopian tubes are open, and we'll see if their uterine cavity is normal.

√ Maintain or Maximize Your Fertility

Some experts believe that the health of the mother matters more than the age of the mother. So make sure you're treating your body like a temple whether you're planning on getting pregnant in the next few months or ten years from now. Plenty of lifestyle factors (smoking, excessive drinking, being overweight) can impact your fertility. You want to be sure to treat any disease that may affect you (like hypertension or diabetes) as well, since that can lead to a high-risk pregnancy. Choose any procedures you have (including fibroid removal and abortions) very carefully so you don't scar your uterus or fallopian tubes.

If you're not planning on getting pregnant anytime soon, you should at least have a conversation with your doctor about the ultimate way to outsmart the clock and maintain your fertility: egg freezing. Learn about what it is, see how much it might cost, and start saving for it if you need to.

If you are planning on getting pregnant, research the latest techniques that can improve your chances of success. You'll hear a lot about everything from eating pineapple to having an orgasm when trying to conceive. But the only proven practices I recommend are taking prenatal vitamins that contain DHA (which can lower your baby's risk of brain and spinal problems), CoQ10 supplements (which may improve the quality of your eggs), and considering acupuncture (which may improve ovarian or follicular function).

√ Practice Safe Sex

Sometimes silent sexually transmitted infections (like chlamydia) can wreak havoc on your reproductive system by scarring your fallopian tubes and more. If you're not with a partner you're in a committed relationship with, use a condom each and every time you have penetrative sex.

√ If You're Not Ready to Conceive, Pick a Birth Control Method (Or Two)

I once had another Mary Jane patient who refused to use birth control. The pill? She said it made her sick and every time she tried it she gained way too much weight. An IUD or the implant? She said she couldn't stand having a foreign substance in her body. The shot? Didn't that cause cancer? This young woman was so misinformed and so uninterested in me setting the record straight. So instead, she kept getting abortions whenever she got pregnant. More than twenty-five terminations, to be exact.

As a physician, I have to say how dangerous this behavior was. Every medical procedure comes with some risk. To willfully submit yourself to dozens of them—unnecessarily—is tempting a terrible fate. She was putting herself at risk for damage to her uterine lining, an infection, or worse. Bottom line: find your perfect contraceptive and you'll never have to worry about waging this level of war over your Queen V.

√ If You're Ready to Conceive, Pick a Method and Watch the Clock

Once again, if you're under thirty-five and have been trying for a year, it's time to get an MD's help. Same for women thirty-five to thirty-nine who have been trying for six months and women over forty who are within the six-month window.

After that six- to twelve-month mark, you want to start thinking about investing in technology (like IUI and IVF, see below) to make your baby dreams come true. You also want to stay woke on what's happening in terms of reproductive technology. When I was trying to get pregnant, egg freezing was an experimental procedure. Nowadays it's a common practice and assisted reproduction is a multibillion-dollar industry. Just a few years ago, for the very first time, a baby was born to a woman who had a uterus transplant. Who knows what may be possible just five to ten years from now?

HOW TO HAVE A BABY:
SO YOU WANT TO BE A MOM?

Any woman who wants to be a mother can usually find a way. Whether you carry a baby forty weeks yourself or let someone else pass you the bassinet through adoption, here's how to be strategic about having a child.

Fertility awareness methods (FAMs) are known as natural family planning, the rhythm method, and, in my book, the original "missionary work." FAMs allow you to know when you're ovulating and most likely to get pregnant. These methods include charting your menstrual cycle on a calendar, taking your temperature orally every day before you get out of bed, and noticing the changes in your cervical mucus. Using multiple FAMs together can work even better, boosting your chances of a baby.

Intrauterine insemination (IUI) is an artificial insemination procedure where sperm is injected through your cervix into your uterus to fertilize an egg. The technique is commonly used with same-sex couples; couples with unexplained fertility problems, low sperm count, or decreased sperm motility; and women with cervical mucus problems. IUI takes place around ovulation, typically twenty-four to thirty-six hours after the hormone that indicates ovulation surges. The short procedure takes place in a clinic or your doctor's office and is usually painless, though some women experience mild cramping. Two weeks after IUI, your doctor or health provider will administer a pregnancy test. IUI isn't recommended for women with a history of pelvic infections, moderate to severe endometriosis, or those who have had severe disease of the fallopian tubes.

In vitro fertilization (IVF) extracts eggs from your ovaries and fertilizes them with sperm in a lab. Embryos develop in a petri dish, and when deemed viable, a doctor inserts them into your uterus for implantation. In some cases, two embryos are transferred at once so with IVF, there's a chance for multiples. One cycle can take about two weeks, and depending on the results, you may need more than one. A single IVF cycle can cost anywhere between $12,000 and $17,000, with an additional cost for medications that typically run from $3,000 to $5,000, and many insurance companies don't cover any IVF costs. Success rates for IVF decrease with age and a woman may have to go through several cycles before becoming pregnant.

Donor eggs make it possible to get pregnant if you can't conceive using your own eggs. An egg donor tends to be a younger woman who provides her eggs to be fertilized with sperm either from the couple's partner or a sperm donor. Once the donor egg and sperm create an embryo in a lab, the recipient undergoes IVF. An egg donor can be anonymous, a family member, or a friend, and she must undergo testing for communicable infectious diseases, genetic screening, and a formal psychological evaluation. Using a donor egg can cost $12,000 to $25,000 or higher.

Surrogacy. After getting pregnant the old-fashioned way, surrogacy is probably next in line for having a centuries-old history. If you're not able to produce an egg yourself or if you're not capable of carrying a baby to full term (perhaps you've had a hysterectomy or have a heart condition), this form of women helping other women start families might be an option for you. Just beware that even though it happens thousands of times a year in the United States, there are a lot of legal strings attached.

There are two types of surrogacy: gestational (in which you use your own egg or a donor egg to create an embryo that the surrogate carries) and traditional (in which you use the surrogate's egg). This isn't an option just for the wealthy. There are altruistic surrogates who go through the process for free, provided that you pay their medical bills. There are also women who are able to ask friends or family members (like a sister or their mother) to carry the child for them. Fees vary depending upon whether the donor is altruistic or not, whether the surrogacy takes place in the United States or abroad, and whether you work with an agency or an independent surrogate. The cost of surrogacy can range from $80,000 to $120,000.

Adoption. One of the biggest decisions you'll have to make once you decide to adopt is whether you will do it abroad or in the United States, either through a public or private agency. After that, another significant consideration is figuring out if you want an open adoption (which allows your child's biological parents to maintain contact) or a closed adoption (where the biological parents stay anonymous).

HOW *NOT* TO HAVE A BABY: SO YOU *DON'T* WANT TO BE A MOM?

Depending upon where you live, there may be no or several options available to you to terminate a pregnancy. Talk with a healthcare provider to figure out next steps, which might include:

Medication abortion is also known as the abortion pill and consists of two different medicines: mifepristone and misoprostol. Mifepristone, taken first, blocks your body's own progesterone, stopping the pregnancy from progressing. Misoprostol can be taken immediately or up to forty-eight hours after mifepristone. It causes cramping and bleeding to empty your uterus and completes the abortion process. The process is similar to having a miscarriage, and you can take the pills in the privacy of your own home. A very effective method, the abortion pill works up to 98 percent of the time on women who are eight to ten weeks pregnant.

Surgical abortion takes place in-clinic or in your doctor's office. The type of procedure depends on how far along you are in your pregnancy. If you're in the first six to sixteen weeks of your pregnancy, you can have a suction abortion or vacuum aspiration. This type uses an instrument to suction the fetus and placenta from the uterus. After sixteen weeks' gestation, a dilation and evacuation (D&E) will be performed. A D&E requires medical tools to remove pregnancy tissue from the uterus, followed by a suction device to make sure the contents are completely removed.

THE SPECIALIST'S CORNER: TEENS AND BIRTH CONTROL

Teen pregnancy rates have declined steadily for the past few decades—hitting an all-time low in 2017. For more than twenty years, Power to Decide, a national nonprofit organization, has worked to support that decline. Through education, work with policymakers, and collaborations with providers, they help women of all ages—and particularly young people—prevent unplanned pregnancies. So I reached out to Ginny Ehrlich, D.Ed, MPH, MS, the chief executive officer of the organization, to talk about how young women are making birth control choices, barriers that still exist to getting access to contraceptives, and what every woman reading this can do to help other women hold on to their power to decide.

Dr. Jackie: Let's talk about that first choice younger women make when it comes to birth control. I know a lot of them just pick what their friends are using or maybe the first thing a provider suggests. But what are some unique ways they should be thinking about that first decision?

> **Dr. Ehrlich:** There is not one answer to this question. Young women should think about whether it matters, for example, if others know that they are on a particular method. Because there are methods that are more hidden, like the shot or the IUD—which is, by the way, fine for teens and young women. And there are methods that are more findable, like birth control pills kept

in your purse. Some methods—like the shot, the IUD, or the implant—don't require any decision-making in the moment, so those may be a better fit if you want a lower-maintenance option. On our organization's website, Bedsider.org, we talk about the different ways young women can think about which method is right for them. Really, the guidance for young people would be to own their bodies and know what's best for their bodies. Your best friend might not like the same music you do or have the same allergies as you—and she may not use the contraceptive method that's also best for you. So it's a matter of doing your research and really understanding what options are out there.

Dr. Jackie: Everyone says life is about the journey, not the destination. But you say that's true of contraception as well and promote the idea of women being on "birth control journeys." What does that mean?

Dr. Ehrlich: It's really meant to recognize and embrace the fact that the average woman spends three decades on some contraceptive method. Clearly life changes during those three decades. In most cases, the method that might be the perfect choice for someone at twenty-two is not necessarily going to work for them at thirty-two, thirty-five, or forty-four. We really like to embrace the fact that it's awesome that there are so many options to switch to on the market because people's lives change, people's bodies change, people's circumstances change, and there's a method for every season of life.

Dr. Jackie: Yes, there are so many options—but I still see a lot of "oops" and "uh-oh" moments in my practice. I also know a lot of women aren't getting the contraceptives they need. Let's tell everyone why.

Dr. Ehrlich: Birth control is not as easy to access as a lot of people think. One issue is the difference between healthcare coverage and healthcare access. Someone can have coverage to support the cost of birth control, but it doesn't mean they have the means or the time to drive hours to the nearest clinic to get a prescription. Also, we know that today about 19.5 million women in need of publicly funded contraception live in what we call "contraceptive deserts." These are counties in which there's not reasonable access to the full range of methods through a public clinic. And "reasonable access" is defined as at least one clinic, or provider, per every *thousand* women in need of publicly funded contraception. To make matters worse, we know that, in addition to those 19.5 million women, there are about 11 million women who have no health insurance, which makes the cost of birth control challenging or out of reach. As policies related to reproductive health change, so do the implications for millions of women.

Dr. Jackie: How can women overcome those financial obstacles and issue of access?

Dr. Ehrlich: We're seeing a really exciting trend with telemedicine companies supporting women to access hormonal methods of contraception without ever visiting a clinic. It's all online. You can use telemedicine "visits" to get prescriptions for hormonal methods, and then have the methods delivered to your door. Right now, there's a new company coming into that marketplace every month. Power to Decide launched our contraceptive access fund, BCBenefits, based on the belief that all women deserve access to birth control. BCBenefits is a digital tool that helps women overcome some of the many barriers, like unreimbursed fees and distance to a clinic, that stand between them and the birth control method of their choice. We're also partnering with telemedicine companies to provide financial assistance for women who can't afford contraceptives through the sites. These aren't the only answers, but they're a start.

Dr. Jackie: Besides knowing their body and advocating for their Queen V, what's one thing you wish every woman would do when it comes to contraception?

Dr. Ehrlich: Knowing yourself and owning your choices—regardless of what other people say. And take care of one another by making sure every woman gets the birth control and the healthcare she needs and deserves. That can be through donations or through advocacy. Let's all do what we can to take care of one another.

THE SPECIALIST'S CORNER: FERTILITY

Whether you're years away from getting pregnant or years past the ability to have babies, this advice from my colleague will change the way you think about fertility forever. Desireé McCarthy-Keith, MD, is an award-winning, board-certified reproductive endocrinologist and regional medical director for Shady Grove Fertility in Atlanta. She's helped thousands of women who have struggled with infertility and she knows that while it can be a lonely battle, we should never make women go it alone. Take her advice to heart on why you need to talk to your doctor about your fertility starting in your twenties, how to find the perfect specialist, and how we all can help other women in their struggle.

Dr. Jackie: So many women think that if they're not ready to have a baby right this second, they don't need to talk to their doctor about their fertility. But we know that's not true. How early is too early to have that talk with your gynecologist?

Dr. McCarthy-Keith: I see fertility patients in their early twenties. You're never too young to have that conversation—but there is a point at which you may be too old. I encourage women to educate themselves and get specific information about their fertility whether they're twenty-five, thirty-five, or forty-five. There are definitely some physicians who will see younger women and say, "Oh, you've got time," and discourage a conversation. But that's a disservice to women.

Dr. Jackie: If your doctor isn't bringing the topic up or shifts the conversation, what should you say? Let's put words in women's mouths.

Dr. McCarthy-Keith: You could say, "I want to get tested to see what my egg reserve is so I know where I stand." Basic bloodwork with your gynecologist can tell you your Anti-Müllerian hormone (AMH) level, which can reveal your ovarian reserve. And an ultrasound can check for any abnormalities of the uterus or ovaries. You could also tell your doctor, "I'm not ready to have a baby yet, but can you tell me about egg freezing?" If you're having an annual exam, that's a perfect opportunity to bring up these questions, address any general fertility concerns, or determine if it's time to see a specialist.

Dr. Jackie: What are the most common reasons that women visit a fertility specialist?

Dr. McCarthy-Keith: Number one would be problems with ovulation, like having PCOS. Many women with PCOS have multiple undeveloped eggs in their ovaries and high testosterone levels, which can lead to irregular menstrual cycles. They may ovulate later in their cycle or not at all from month to month. Second would be abnormalities of the uterus, like fibroids, which impact 70 percent of women by the time we reach menopause, or blocked fallopian tubes. Third would be declining egg reserve due to advanced age. I would add a bonus reason to the list: male factor. We see sperm abnormalities either exclusively or in addition to a female factor in up to 40 percent of couples who are having trouble conceiving.

Dr. Jackie: If you're having trouble getting pregnant, how do you find the best infertility specialist for your particular problem?

> **Dr. McCarthy-Keith:** Make a list of fertility clinics in your area, paying attention to their success rates and patient reviews online. Read about the services they offer and research any special interests their providers have. If you have a unique situation, you want to meet with a physician who has expertise in the area you're struggling with. There are many providers who have special training in dealing with uterine fibroids, endometriosis, or PCOS. They see more of those types of patients, may have more extensive training, and may have done more current research in that area. Prior to scheduling a visit, research general costs for treatments and find out which services are covered by insurance and which would be out of pocket for you.

Dr. Jackie: What do you wish more women knew about meeting with a specialist?

> **Dr. McCarthy-Keith:** That they should feel empowered—not embarrassed—when they make that first appointment. Building a family truly takes a village. But often women are frustrated, ashamed, defensive, or sad that they have not conceived on their own. Those feelings can sometimes get in the way of them having a productive visit.

Dr. Jackie: As you may know, I became infertile after cancer treatments to fight breast cancer back in 2004. Any advice to women who might face a similar battle today?

> **Dr. McCarthy-Keith:** Women have more options now for family building after cancer than they ever have before. There is usually a small window of a few weeks from cancer diagnosis to starting chemotherapy where women can harvest their eggs

before they are exposed to the chemotherapy. Egg freezing can be accomplished over a two- to three-week period, and then those eggs can be safely stored until a woman is cancer-free and ready to get pregnant. Some women will choose to carry a pregnancy from an egg donor or adopt a child to fulfill their dream of having a family after cancer treatment.

Dr. Jackie: What *aren't* people talking about when it comes to infertility that you wish they were saying more about?

Dr. McCarthy-Keith: Many people *aren't* talking about infertility at all. We need to remove the stigma associated with infertility. This is a common medical condition—just like heart disease or diabetes—that affects 7.5 million women and their partners every year. We have to chip away at the idea that it's an anomaly by normalizing the conversation around it. Everyone can talk about it. And the more women, like you, are willing to share their experiences with it publicly, the easier it will be to reshape everyone's perception of what infertility is. We can all work to get rid of the stigma.

THE SPECIALIST'S CORNER: ABORTIONS

One in four women will have an abortion by the time they reach their forty-fifth birthday. That's a lot of women for an issue that rarely gets discussed. So I'm discussing it here. As I mentioned early on, this book is for everyone and I want to provide information that applies to everyone. So when I was looking for an expert who could offer some insight on the procedure, I turned to Jamila Perritt, MD, MPH, former medical director at Planned Parenthood and a family planning and reproductive health specialist who provides care in Washington, DC, Maryland, and Virginia. Whether you're for or against the procedure, she has invaluable knowledge and over a decade of experience to share in our "V" Q&A about who *really* gets abortions, the most important question to ask yourself if you're considering one, what an abortion doula is, and more.

Dr. Jackie: The fact that one in four women will have an abortion is going to shock a lot of people.

> **Dr. Perritt:** True, but think of it this way: most Americans say that they want one or two children. So that means people with the ability to get pregnant spend a really short portion of their life either trying to get pregnant, being pregnant, or being postpartum. The rest of the time—about thirty years of their life—they're trying to *prevent* pregnancy. The likelihood of having an unintended pregnancy over a thirty-year time period is pretty high.

Dr. Jackie: Sure! Three decades is a pretty long time.

> **Dr. Perritt:** Yes. Despite the fact that almost half of all pregnancies are unintended, one of the most common statements people make when they come to see me because they have an unintended pregnancy they don't want to or can't carry to term is: "I never thought I would be in this position to make this decision," or "I can't believe this happened to me."

Dr. Jackie: Can you explain to everyone the most common ways people have abortions?

> **Dr. Perritt:** In the United States, abortions can be done either using medication or using a suction procedure. The suction abortion is the one people think of most commonly. A lot of people aren't aware that medication abortion is an option.

Dr. Jackie: You talk about the fact that there's a myth around the particular type of woman who has an abortion. Who do people think she is?

    Dr. Perritt: Someone who is irresponsible, careless, lazy. But the truth is that all kinds of individuals have abortions. These are our mothers, our sisters, and our friends. There's no separation along racial or ethnic lines or income levels. But there are inequities and disparities. That has to do with unequal access to care in certain communities. Communities with higher rates of unintended pregnancy also have higher rates of abortion. And it's these folks that have to walk through protesters at the abortion clinic. But those with access to private doctors and health insurance have their abortions in secret and aren't shamed or stigmatized in the same way.

Dr. Jackie: How are people working to destigmatize abortions?

    Dr. Perritt: I've seen movement recently around abortion storytelling as a way to push back on stigma and shame. So whether we're talking about #wetestify or #shoutyourabortion, there are folks saying, "Listen, this is not uncommon. We're not women of ill repute. This is a common procedure. It's a safe procedure. And this situation happens to many of us."

Dr. Jackie: You said some communities have higher rates of unintended pregnancy because of decreased access. Is that the only issue or are other things at play here?

    Dr. Perritt: For those who have access to birth control but don't want to use it, mistrust of the medical community and of contraception in general is often a factor. In many communities, the historical legacy of reproductive oppression and abuse in this country factors into the decision-making process. Just google James Marion Sims—whom people call the father of modern gynecology—and his research on black slaves without anesthesia. Or look up the unethical birth control experiments on women in Puerto Rico in the 1950s. All of that is what people bring into the office when I say, "What do you want to use for birth control?" and they say, "Nothing," or "I'm against birth control."

Dr. Jackie: What's the most important question you could ask if you're considering having an abortion?

> **Dr. Perritt:** "How easy or difficult will it be for me to access this care when and if I need it?" That brings you to two more questions you need to ask. The first is: "Does my healthcare provider do abortions?" And that's an important one because if you're living in a state with restrictions to access to care, it's going to be infinitely difficult for you to get the care you need. The second is: "Does my insurance cover it?" If you have government-sponsored insurance, the answer is probably no. If you have a small employer-sponsored insurance plan, the answer is probably no. Although abortion is safe and legal, these barriers make it inaccessible to many people.

Dr. Jackie: I hope my patients know they can turn to me for advice around this, but I know not every woman feels this way. How do most women find an abortion provider?

> **Dr. Perritt:** It can be difficult. I once saw a woman who had four kids and was on her fifth pregnancy. She came to see me because her OB-GYN—who was a friend of the family—and her husband were celebrating her pregnancy, but she was consumed with dread. She couldn't take a fifth baby. If you're unable or unwilling to carry your pregnancy to term, I would hope you'd be able to talk to your provider. But I don't think that most people do. I think most start with their insurance

or an independent clinic in their community. The shame and stigma that surround abortion lead people to automatically go outside their provider. A lot of folks I talk to express explicit concern that their doctor will find out they had an abortion. They ask me, "Will my doctor be able to tell when I get back?"

Dr. Jackie: Are there any emotional questions you need to ask yourself before you have an abortion?

   Dr. Perritt: Yes! "What kind of emotional support do I want or need in the decision-making process and following care?" In DC, we have a wonderful community of abortion doulas. These are folks who are solely dedicated to providing emotional support for individuals who want it or need it during their abortion process. I don't want to craft it like it's emotional turmoil for everyone. Some individuals don't want this as part of their process. But for those who want it and need it, find out how you can can seek those services. It's a wonderful way to move through the space with dignity, agency, and support.

POINT OF V: BEING WOKE ISN'T JUST FOR POLITICS

Over the course of the two or three decades that we're fertile, every woman falls into one of three categories: women who are actively trying to get pregnant, women who are actively making sure they don't get pregnant, and women who are keeping their fingers crossed (but not their legs). I'm a firm believer in the power of prayer, but it's not a form of birth control—and neither is hoping or wishing. Raising a child isn't as easy (or hilarious) as it looks on television shows and in movies. And just because your friends and family aren't talking about their struggle with infertility, doesn't mean that it doesn't hurt them. Finding peace with infertility has taken me a lot of time and required a lot of prayer. But recalling memories just to write this chapter was like ripping a scab right off a wound that had been healed so many years ago. However, I believe in always taking my miseries and creating a ministry. If this chapter does one thing, I want it to encourage you to stay woke when it comes to your fertility. Figure out how to prevent pregnancy if that's not what you want, how to stay fertile if you do, and how to use technology to your advantage if you are having trouble conceiving. And if motherhood isn't in your future, know that you don't have to stop living your life because you can't carry your own child. There are so many creative ways to become a mother without birthing a child. I find joy in them every day and I know you will too.

Stop with the Déjà Vu Appointments

THE PROBLEM WITH GETTING COMFORTABLE BEING UNCOMFORTABLE

One of the most powerful motivational mantras I've heard in a long time is a reminder to get comfortable being uncomfortable. If you want to move forward at your job, you need to be able to deal with uncomfortable situations like asking your supervisor for feedback or sweating your way through a presentation to the whole office. (Hey, they call it "work" for a reason.) If you want to strengthen your relationships, you have to be able to handle uncomfortable conversations when your partner has let you down or when you've let them down. And if you want to improve your health, you have to deal with being uncomfortable sporting spandex or dragging yourself to the gym. If you can get comfortable with uncomfortable moments like these, you'll be happy, healthy, and wealthy . . . most of the time.

As positive as that mantra is, there's a problem when people take it too far. Sometimes women get comfortable with a level of discomfort that never goes away. I've had patients get comfortable with fibroids that make them bleed so heavily they get lightheaded around their period. Or overactive bladders that mean they're never sleeping through the night because they keep getting up to go to the bathroom. Or sex so painful that their partner is more of a roommate than a husband. None of these are symptoms I want you to get comfortable with. They're symptoms to confront head-on. They're an SOS from your body to your brain saying, first, "Something's wrong!" and second, "You need to fix this!"

But almost every day I see everyone from Virgin Marys to Notorious V.A.G.s who have gotten complacent in their pain. They come in to see me, tell me all about how they're managing the excessive bleeding by only wearing black pants during their period—but ooh, did they have a close call last week at work. Or that they've gotten used to not getting a good night's sleep and that's why they're so tired at our appointment right now. Or that they don't miss sex so much anyway but boy is their husband giving them a hard time.

They don't want to cure the problem because they've developed work-arounds for the symptoms. Or so they think. They finish our appointment, go home, and come back to me next year with the same complaints. Just worse. That fibroid has gone from the size of a lemon to a grapefruit. They didn't go on that car trip with their family because they were worried about access to bathrooms. Their husband has started complaining loudly about not having sex.

These are the meetings I call déjà vu appointments because when I walk in, I get that feeling we've had this conversation before. And one look at your chart proves it.

"You told me about this last year and the year before and the year before that," I'll say to my déjà vu patients to try to nudge them in the direction of action. "Now, are you sharing these symptoms with me as an FYI or do you want to do something about them?"

It's tough love. But it's still love. I want your Queen V sitting on her throne, not laid out sick in bed. I want you to feel whole and happy. But for that to happen, you need to take action sooner when it's easier to fix the problem. Not later—when it's an emergency situation and much harder to get you back to normal. Unfortunately, so many women don't take action until they get to a breaking point. Those fibroids get so large they're preventing you from getting pregnant—or may be the culprit of a miscarriage. Your overactive bladder led to an embarrassing accident at the office. Decreased intimacy is causing a rift in your marriage.

Ladies, don't wait for a breakdown to move you to a breakthrough. Your wounds are not your fault—but your healing is your responsibility. I know it's not easy. But the hardest part is making the mental decision that you are willing to do what it takes to repair, rebuild, and restore your Queen V so she can go back on her pedestal. Once you're ready and willing, you just need to be able. There are a few F-words that hold us back from that ability—instead of propelling us forward. But here's how you can overcome them.

BREAKING THROUGH BARRIERS TO BETTER HEALTH

Your Finances

My desire is for women to be able to live by choice—not by chance. But sometimes our cash flow has more control over our choices than we'd like it to. If you're worried that a procedure is too expensive and your insurance won't cover it, the first thing you have to do is find out for sure. Some of us walk into a clothing store and won't even look at the price tag of an item we like because we can tell it costs more than we can afford. (Truth be told, sometimes we don't walk into the store at all because we think it's out of our price range.) But there's no charge for looking. The same goes for healthcare.

Call your insurance company or work with a healthcare advocate to figure out the real cost of a procedure. If you don't have insurance, talk to the finance department at your doctor's office and see if they can offer you a discount for paying out of pocket. Ask your doctor, search online, or talk to friends and coworkers and get recommendations for reputable and affordable clinics nearby that provide services on a sliding scale. If you're open to different types of treatment options, ask your doctor about or look online to find clinical trials in your area. I've started offering clinical trials to patients at my office. The beauty is that the trial organizers pay for everything—sometime including the cost of you getting to my office.

I can't tell you how to spend your money, but I can ask you to crunch the numbers. Calculate how much cash you lose every month when you call in sick because your period has you stuck in bed. Honestly, think about how expensive divorce is when you partner decides they're not comfortable being uncomfortable, like you, and they want out. Health problems can hit your wallet when you don't do anything about them. When you look at it this way, maybe you can't afford to ignore them any longer.

Your Fears

I once had a Mary Jane patient who déjà vu'd me for years over her fibroids. Periods lasting two weeks? Yes. Lower back pain? Absolutely. Constantly going to the bathroom because the tumors were pressing on her bladder? Mm-hmm. But she didn't want to do anything about them because she was afraid of losing her uterus and becoming infertile. By the time she said yes to surgery, it was too late. I tried to preserve her uterus, but I had to remove over 100 fibroids. Plus, she was reaching the age where her ovaries weren't willing to release an egg.

Sometimes we're so busy trying to avoid the thing we're afraid of that we end up running right into it. Yes, you can lose your uterus if something goes wrong during a surgery. But you can also lose your uterus if you ignore a problem and don't have surgery, like my Mary Jane patient. Fear limits you—and your vision of your best self. Don't let your worries wear on you so much that you don't explore your best options with your doctor.

Now, I want to make sure you hear me: this is definitely about exploring your options—of which there are almost always more than one. I never try to talk a patient into surgery. There are plenty of ways to treat fibroids that don't involve anesthesia. I don't do convincing. I simply present the facts and let you decide which path—medication? an IUD? surgery?—is right for you. The worst thing a patient can do is have surgery and have remorse. I want you to be at peace with whatever choice you make for positive change. You are the CMO (Chief Medical Officer) for your health.

Your Fantasy

You can be ready to take action but still be hoping, wishing and praying for the problem to go away by alternative means. You know what I'm talking about, ladies. Drinking green tea and popping chasteberry pills. Eating more veggies and swearing off alcohol. Trying that mystery remedy your cousin's coworker's friend heard about online. Now, some of these things actually work—but they're treating the symptoms—not eliminating the problem entirely. When you're talking about fibroids, some alternative methods can make the fibroid harder to remove during surgery because they may soften its texture. Talk with your doctor about the path of action you're choosing and how it may impact you down the line.

Your First Diagnosis

I had a woman with adenomyosis who was in tears after finally getting the right diagnosis, telling me, "I was hurting, I was in pain, but nobody believed me!" The people you give power to have power over you. So make sure whoever is on your healthcare team deserves their spot. One way to do that is by getting comfortable being uncomfortable when you say the following six words: "Can I get a second opinion?" Two MDs can be better than one. Consulting more than one professional—especially when we're talking about surgery—is not just reassuring. It's also a smart way to get rid of all those other barriers we just talked about. Your second opinion doctor might know of a free clinical trial your first one didn't, or he or she might do a better job calming your fears or know more about why your fantasy treatment just won't pan out. Hearing the same thing twice will also reassure you that the treatment options are right for you. Medical advice doesn't have to be a one-and-done approach. You owe it to your Queen V to do your research.

6 COMMON DÉJÀ VU CONDITIONS

With every déjà vu appointment, you're getting further away from the Queen V of a thriving nation and closer to a Queen V of a war-torn country just trying to hold it together. You might not even recognize the woman you've become, the workarounds you've adopted, and the lengths you've gone to get through the day. So I'll help you spot the patterns—and get your Queen V back to happier, healthier times.

Do you recognize this woman? "Supersize" tampons don't cut it because you can feel blood gush right past them long before the four-hour mark. You've put up with the misery of handwashing blood out of your underwear, pants, and bed sheets. You're exercising like crazy but can't seem to trim your waist. When someone asks you out for dinner or to visit their house, you check your calendar . . . to see if you'll be on your period and popping Advil like candy. If that sounds familiar, you might have . . .

. . . **fibroids**, benign growths that appear in the uterus, on the outer surface of the uterine wall, or within the uterine wall in up to 80 percent of women by age fifty. While you may not notice them, your doctor can feel them during a pelvic exam or see them on an ultrasound. I once had a beautiful young woman cock her head and look at me in shock when I told her I could feel her fibroids. She shot back, "Who has fibroids?" "You do," I said. I ordered an ultrasound so we could both see the markedly enlarged mass that ended up being a little bigger than a grapefruit. Fibroids vary in number—some women just have one, and that Mary Jane I told you about had over 100. They can also vary in size. These muscular tumors can be a small seedling or a gigantic mass keeping you from buttoning up your skinny jeans. If you've never had a baby, your uterus is no bigger than your fist. But I've seen fibroids that made a woman look like she was carrying a nine-pound baby. When that happens, none of your other organs have the room or capacity to function in the way they're supposed to and the fibroids can cause urinary incontinence or constipation. You're basically allowing one organ to control the house.

Some lucky women out there have fibroids but not a single symptom to go with them. These aren't the déjà vu appointments I'm worried about.

It's everyone else who experiences heavy bleeding during menstruation; periods lasting more than a week; pelvic pain or pressure; backaches or leg pains; or an enlarged abdomen. It's everyone else who is having difficulty getting pregnant and putting their baby at risk because of these tumors. My partner once performed surgery on a Sanctified Snatch who thought she was having twins. But an ultrasound was performed and she could see a fifty-centimeter fibroid that was bigger than the twenty-four-week-old baby. During surgery, the doctor had to pull out the uterus (yes, with the baby inside it), remove the fibroid, and put the uterus right back in the patient's abdomen. Moral of the story: prenatal care is so important, ladies. Get any fibroids taken care of before you get pregnant.

Thankfully, you have a few treatment options, including fibroid-shrinking hormonal drugs. There are also several different types of surgical procedures, including a hysteroscopic myomectomy (surgery to remove the growths through the vagina), laparoscopic myomectomy (surgery done with minimal incisions through your abdomen), or open myomectomy (using a C-section-type incision through your abdomen). There is also uterine artery embolization (which is also minimally invasive and cuts off blood supply to the fibroid but may not be ideal if you want to get pregnant later). If other treatments haven't worked or aren't appropriate, a hysterectomy may also be an option.

> **Do you recognize this woman?** You're used to curling up in a ball from excruciating period pain that feels like knives stabbing at your abdomen. You've missed days of work (there was no way you'd be able to make it out of bed, much less make it in) from the heavy periods and the shooting pain. You've been trying to get pregnant, but it's just not working and doctors aren't sure why. If any of this sounds familiar, you might have . . .
>
> **. . . endometriosis or adenomyosis.** Let's start off talking about endometriosis, which occurs when the endometrium (the inner lining of the uterus) grows outside the uterus and on other areas such as the ovaries, fallopian tubes, bowel, bladder, and the outer surface of the uterus. I've seen endometriosis spread as far as the vagina,

the belly button, and the lungs. With endometriosis, your uterine lining continues to thicken, break down, and bleed when you menstruate. But because it's outside the uterus, the displaced tissue becomes trapped with no place to go. Also, when the lining gets outside your uterus, the body recognizes it as foreign and starts to attack it. The result: swelling, inflammation, and intense chronic pain in your abdomen, lower back, pelvis, and legs. Infertility and digestive problems are common as well.

The craziest thing is that people who are in the most pain from this disease can tend to have the least scar tissue noted surgically. I may see one little tiny spot of endometriosis when I look inside them. But those who have the least pain can have the worst disease. I'll look inside them with a laparoscope and say, "What in the world?" The scar tissue is everywhere.

It may take up to several years for a woman to get diagnosed with endometriosis—which is more common in women in their thirties and forties. Part of the problem is that the best way to diagnose endometriosis is to put your eyes on it. Ultrasounds and MRIs can show me *some* of what's happening inside you, but there's no misdiagnosing endometriosis if I happen to see it with my naked eye while I'm doing a tubal ligation, an ovarian cystectomy, or a diagnostic laparoscopy. Sometimes endometriosis makes your abdomen look like a haunted house, with raw, ragged, black adhesions hanging from different organs. Other times it looks as if someone poured cement inside your abdomen and shook it up.

Without a cause, it's hard to have a cure. And we don't know why more than 6.5 million women in the US have endometriosis. One theory is that it's retrograde bleeding back into your abdomen that happens with your period. Another is that some women were simply born with cells outside their uterus prone to growing this tissue. Regardless of the cause, our best treatment includes birth control pills, pain medications, and in severe cases, surgery to cut or burn away adhesions. Lifestyle modifications can help too, like acupuncture (it's been shown to reduce endo pain) or cutting back on red meat (which can increase inflammation).

Adenomyosis and endometriosis are basically first cousins. Adeno-myosis happens when the inner lining of the uterus grows into its mus-cular wall, at times causing the uterus to enlarge to two to three times its normal size. (Think of adenomyosis as endometriosis that only happens on the inside walls of your uterus.) Because of where the disease presents itself, it's a hard diagnosis. Transvaginal ultrasounds and MRIs can give us an idea of what's going on inside the walls of your uterus, but we really don't see it until someone has a surgery. I once had a young patient who we thought had ovarian cancer. It wasn't until I was in the operating room with her that we realized there were no tumors, no fibroids, just adeno-myomas wreaking havoc on her abdomen.

To be clear, adenomyosis is a benign disorder—but it doesn't always feel that way because it can cause all the same frustrating and agonizing symptoms that endometriosis can: painful, heavy periods; abnormal uter-ine bleeding; and chronic pelvic pain. It's also rarely talked about—even though it may impact up to 65 percent of women. The hush-hush around it is probably tied to the fact we don't know why it happens. Some theories point to uterine inflammation after childbirth (women who have more than one child are at higher risk), previous surgical procedures on your uterus causing inflammation, or simply being born that way.

Unfortunately, we don't know how to cure adenomyosis either. Unlike fibroids, which I can peel off like an orange peel, adenomyosis spreads like ivy in the walls of your uterus. We can only treat the pain you feel from it—not remove it. So, really, this is a déjà vu appointment because science hasn't come up with a solution yet. Treatments include anti-inflammatory drugs, hormone medication (like birth control pills or Lupron), or in extreme cases, a hysterectomy. Time can heal this wound: most cases occur in women in their forties and fifties (but experts aren't sure if that's due to late diagnoses or not), and adenomyomas usually resolve themselves after menopause.

Do you recognize this woman? You've stopped wearing tampons because for some reason they're just too painful to get inside you.

You've been convincing your partner to have a lot more oral sex (which, honestly, isn't that hard) because vaginal penetration is way too painful for you. While your partner is snoring away after sex, you're awake because your vagina is throbbing with pain—even though you had sex hours ago. If any of this sounds familiar, you might have . . .

. . . **dyspareunia**. It's basically a big blanket term for persistent vaginal pain during and even after intercourse. Between 10 and 20 percent of women in the United States experience this condition and the list of reasons why is endless. If I put them all here, it would sound like the list of side effects rattled off during a drug commercial. That just means that it will take you working with your doctor to get to the bottom of the problem. Most doctors will start by listening to your medical history, getting a sense of your other symptoms, and doing a physical exam. You can help them by being as specific as possible in answering their questions: Does it hurt as soon as your partner enters you or only with deep penetration? Is it on one side more than the other? Are you in pain when you're not having sex? What makes it better? What makes the pain worse? Have you experienced any recent trauma to your vagina?

Your answers can help us narrow down the possible causes and then try to diagnose your pain through a process of elimination: If you're only in pain while having sex and lubricant makes sex less painful, then your problem may be vaginal dryness, which can come from taking birth control pills or transitioning into menopause. If you've been in constant pain and have a discharge, I can do a culture and find out you've got an infection.

When I've eliminated all the physical reasons for painful sex but you still can't bear penetration, then we have to talk about emotional ones. Psychological problems are the leading cause of dyspareunia. Let's be clear: I don't mean that the issue is all in your head. You're truly in pain, whether you're a Virgin Mary with a fear of intimacy, a Coochie-Chondriac with tight pelvic floor muscles due to stress, a Sanctified Snatch with body image issues, a Mary Jane in an unhappy marriage, or a Notorious V.A.G. dealing with a past sexual trauma like rape or molestation. Yes, you're in pain, but I can't fix it. So I'll refer you to a therapist who may offer nonmedication treatments like vaginal relaxation exercises, counseling, or sex therapy.

> **Do you recognize this woman?** You've stopped wearing tampons because they feel like they're going to fall out—or actually do. You've noticed blood in your underwear from skin rubbing up against the fabric. You feel pressure, like something is bulging outside your vagina, but if you ignore it, it's not so bad. You've had a leakage accident before or bowel movements that are a real struggle. And there was that one time you pushed on your genitals to empty your bowels. If any of this sounds familiar, you might have . . .
>
> . . . **pelvic organ prolapse**, where your organs are no longer being supported by muscle or tissue inside you and begin to drop down in your body and into your vaginal canal. Prolapse can occur in different parts of your abdomen—causing your bladder or uterus to descend into your vagina, or your intestines or rectum to push into your vagina. One of the worst cases of prolapse I've ever seen was a Sanctified Snatch whose entire uterus was hanging out of the vagina. I'm not sure how she was able to walk into my office being in that much pain. Despite the fact that she didn't have good health insurance, she was at her breaking point.

Pelvic organ prolapse impacts about 3 percent of American women but often goes underdiagnosed because many physicians aren't familiar with the different types of prolapse that exist. (They're categorized by the pelvic organ impacted, from your uterus to your intestines.) Vaginal childbirth (especially if your baby weighed over 8.5 pounds), persistent pressure on your abdomen (from being obese or having a chronic cough), or simply getting older can put you at risk for this disorder. But there are plenty of options to heal yourself, including pelvic floor therapy (see Principle #2), having your doctor insert a pessary (usually a disc-shaped plastic or silicone device to offer physical support), or surgery to strengthen the pelvic floor.

> **Do you recognize this woman?** You try not to laugh too much when you're at the movies or hanging out with friends because it makes you pee a little when you do. Before you leave the house, you make note of where all the public bathrooms are on your route in case you need to make a stop. You wear pantyliners even when you don't have your period. You usually wake up tired because you've gotten up a few times in the middle of the night to go to the bathroom. Ride a rollercoaster with your kid? No way, no how. If any of this sounds familiar, you might have . . .
>
> **. . . urinary incontinence.** A lot of women think that having to go to the bathroom all the time is just part of getting older or that it's just one of those things that happens with everyone after a baby, so it's fine. Nope. That ain't right. Sure, it's common: twenty-five million American adults suffer from some form of urinary incontinence. But it's not normal. And for the record, it happens to women who haven't ever given birth too.

Incontinence occurs when unexpected muscle spasms or pressure on your bladder (which can come from coughing, sneezing, laughing, or being overweight) cause you to leak urine.

If this is a once in a blue moon kind of thing for you, then you probably just need to watch your alcohol or caffeine intake. Both substances can increase your chances of an accident. But if you're organizing your life around access to bathrooms, it's time to talk to your doctor about your options, which include pelvic floor physical therapy (see Principle #2), inserting a pessary (either through your doctor or purchasing one over the counter), a collagen injection, or surgery.

EVERY WOMAN NEEDS THESE 4 PEOPLE ON HER SEXUAL HEALTH TEAM

I preach the gospel of advocating for your health, but it doesn't have to be a one-woman job. There are plenty of people around you who can support you in getting the premium care that your Queen V deserves. Here's who should be in your fave four:

Your OB-GYN. Surprise, surprise. Yes, I want you going to your doctor like clockwork for your regular well-woman visits. But not just any doctor. Get a doctor you feel comfortable with, one who gives you his or her full attention when you're in the room and you can say anything to without feeling judged. Then do it! Say anything. Ask about anal sex, your one-night stand, switching to a better birth control to help with your acne, dealing with painful intercourse, your adulterous affair, or how you can get gender reassignment surgery. Tell them if you've ever been sexually assaulted or suffered any type of trauma so they're aware of any physical or emotional repercussions that may pop up. Or just take a second on the exam table to ask, "Does everything look normal down there?"

I once saw a twelve-year-old girl whose mother brought her in. Mom was freaking out because she thought something was wrong with her daughter's vulva. It turned out her vaginal flower was a blossoming peace lily—one labium was barely there and the other side was very prominent. I was able to explain to the daughter that she was normal and make her feel okay about her anatomy. While I strongly recommended she not have intercourse until she was much older, I also suggested that when she did, she talk to her partner about what her vagina looks like so he or she would be prepared. This little lady could've been destined to become a Coochie-Chondriac from her mother making her so worried about her anatomy. But our conversation may have nudged her to another VP.

Your BFF. She's good for more than just shaking her head back and forth when you complain about your lying, cheating ex. Sometimes, it's a good girlfriend who explains to you that what you think is normal (a period that lasts ten days) is really a problem you need to get checked out already. She can also be the one who talks a Coochie-Chondriac out of booking a third appointment because she's positive she has a vaginal infection. (A good girlfriend will confirm, "Girl, get over that. I don't smell nothing you need to worry about.") She's the Notorious V.A.G. who can tell you about the incredible new condom you have to try out or the Mary Jane who offers to go to an appointment with you if you're nervous.

My Virgin Marys and Sanctified Snatches have sexual secrets they'll be taking to the grave, so I know it's going to be hard to convince them to bare all to a bestie. They're prim, proper, and not about to profess what happens when they're in a paper gown or behind the bathroom or bedroom door. But it's worth reconsidering that mind-set. You're missing out on a wealth of information from your friends. Maybe start with small details (like your PMS symptoms or your curiosity about vajacials) rather than big ones (like which vaginal flower you are or which STIs you've had).

Your partner. If your significant other isn't helping you tend to your Queen V, you're in trouble. Who better to tell you that the waxing salon you're going to isn't really doing you any favors? Or that it's way past time to do something about your period pain because s/he can't stand seeing you doubled over every month? I'll be honest: it took me a long time to get to the point where I felt comfortable being open and honest with my husband about my periods and vaginal odor. But once I did it was liberating.

Your therapist. You don't know how mucked up in the head you might be until you talk to someone who can show you the city line between normal town and crazy town. I came from a very sheltered background and didn't realize how many sexual hangups I had until I got married. Even if you only go to a therapist one time, those forty-five minutes might completely change your life.

ACT LIKE A LADY, THINK LIKE AN MD

Sometimes I walk into the exam room and feel like a stopwatch has just clicked. I don't want to make anyone sitting in the waiting room restless, but I also want to spend as much time with my patients as possible, so I'm racing against the clock. If you come to your appointment prepared to answer most of the questions I'm going to ask, we can knock out your routine exam, get to the bottom of any problems you're having, and still have time for me to answer your extra questions about organic tampons or laser hair removal. Here's how to prep for your meeting like a pro:

- Be able to tell me the date when your last period started without hesitation. No fumbling for your phone or staring confused at the calendar on my wall. (C'mon. You know I'm going to ask. Every single time. So just look it up in the waiting room.)
- Cover the five Ws (and an H) of any problem you're having. For example, if it's pelvic pain:
  - ✦ Who are you having sex with? (Is there a new partner or are you not using condoms?)
  - ✦ What makes the pain better or worse?
  - ✦ When was the last time it hurt? (I need a date, not you saying, "A while ago.")
  - ✦ Where do you feel the pain?
  - ✦ How much does it hurt on a scale of 1 to 10? (Is it a dull ache? Stabbing or shooting?)
  - ✦ Why do you think it's happening? (Did you have some crazy sex last weekend? Are you taking any herbal supplements?)

- Tell me if you're keeping secrets. If your partner doesn't know that you got herpes last year after a one-night stand (instead of years ago in college like you told them), I need a heads-up. I see tons of women who have not revealed their HSV status. I specifically remember a Sanctified Snatch who asked for an elective C-section to prevent any possible transmission of herpes to her baby. She asked me to not share her reasoning with her husband. Then she decided to reveal all on the operating table. She left me looking like a bald-faced liar!

- Watch the clock. For all the patients who like a good girlfriend doctor they can kiki it up with, please don't complain about having to spend a long time in the waiting room. Remember that I am your doctor first and foremost. I can't stay in the exam room with you forever talking about what happened on the show last night. So let's address your health concerns. Trust me, I'm not going to rush you along.

POINT OF V: TAKE ACTION!

The definition of insanity is doing the same thing over and over again—but expecting a different outcome. My déjà vu patients are coming to the office for their appointments and complaining about the same symptoms over and over again—but they don't accept the outcome will always be the same until they take action. I can't stop your bladder leakage from embarrassing you on the train if you won't let me help you. I can't stop you from going down the path to a sexless marriage if you won't let us do something about your pain. No matter how busy, broke, or scared you might be, where there's a will there's a way. Help me to help you get your Queen V to her healthiest state.

BIBLIOGRAPHY

This book is the culmination of my training and decades of practice and experience as a physician wearing a white coat. But I also pulled information from interviews with experts, trusted medical sources, health research, and online articles. To keep things interesting, I turned to my Instagram following as well to get a sense of what women across the world who don't come to my office are experiencing. I've done my best in this section to provide sources for all content that didn't come directly from me.

INTRODUCTION

On *Fifty Shades of Grey*:
Acuna, Kirsten, "By the Numbers: The 'Fifty Shades of Grey' Phenomenon," *Business Insider*, September 4, 2013.
"The Top-Earning Authors of 2013," Forbes.com.

PRINCIPLE #1: DON'T CALL IT WRONG IF YOU DON'T KNOW WHAT'S RIGHT

General background on female anatomy:
Knudtson, Jennifer, "Female External Genital Organs," Merck Manuals.
    "What Are the Parts of the Female Sexual Anatomy?" Planned Parenthood.
Leelo, Jamie, "The 5 Types of Vaginas, as Revealed by a Bikini Waxer," Elite Daily, April 4, 2017.
Scaccia, Annamarya, author, and Holly Ernst, PA-C, medical reviewer, "Lopsided Vagina: Are My Labia Normal?" Healthline, June 6, 2018.
Thomason, Kristine, "10 Things You Never Knew About the Clitoris," Health, June 29, 2017.

General resources for information on vaginal problems:
Michigan Medicine at the University of Michigan, www.uofmhealth.org.
American Academy of Dermatology, www.aad.org.

American Cancer Society, www.cancer.org.

American College of Obstetrics and Gynecology, www.acog.org.

Mayo Clinic, www.mayoclinic.org.

On douching:

Eschenbach, David A., Soe Soe Thwin, Dorothy L. Patton, Thomas M. Hooton, Ann E. Stapleton, Kathy Agnew, Carol Winter, Amalia Meier, and Walter E. Stamm, "Influence of the Normal Menstrual Cycle on Vaginal Tissue, Discharge, and Microflora," *Clinical Infectious Diseases* 30(6), June 2000, 901–7.

Hay, Phillip E., "Bacterial Vaginosis as a Mixed Infection," in Kim A. Brogden and Janet M. Guthmiller, eds., *Polymicrobial Diseases*, Washington, DC: ASM Press, 2002, 200.

U.S. Department of Health & Human Services, Office on Women's Health, www.womenshealth.gov.

On labiaplasty:

Horton, Karen, "Stats Show Labiaplasty Is Becoming More Popular," American Society of Plastic Surgeons, April 25, 2017, www.plasticsurgery.org/news/blog/stats-show -labiaplasty-is-becoming-more-popular.

PRINCIPLE #2: VAJACIALS ARE REAL—BUT YOU ONLY NEED ONE THING FOR DOWN THERE CARE

On vaginal bacteria and UTIs:

Gilbert, Nicole M., Valerie P. O'Brien, and Amanda L. Lewis, "Transient Microbiota Exposures Activate Dormant *Escherichia coli* Infection in the Bladder and Drive Severe Outcomes of Recurrent Disease," *PLOS Pathogens* 13(3), March 30, 2017.

On douching:

Branch, Francesca, Tracey J. Woodruff, Susanna D. Mitro, and Ami R. Zota, "Vaginal Douching and Racial/Ethnic Disparities in Phthalates Exposures Among Reproductive-Aged Women: National Health and Nutrition Examination Survey 2001–2004," *Environmental Health* 14(1), 2015.

Martino, Jenny L. and Sten H. Vermund, "Vaginal Douching: Evidence for Risks or Benefits to Women's Health," *Epidemiologic Reviews* 24(2), February 2002, 109–24.

U.S. Department of Health & Human Services, Office on Women's Health, www.womenshealth.gov.

On asparagus and bodily fluids:

Markt, Sarah C., Elizabeth Nuttall, Constance Turman, Jennifer Sinnott, Eric B. Rimm, Ethan Ecsedy, Robert H. Unger, Katja Fall, Stephen Finn, Majken K. Jensen, Jennifer R. Rider, Peter Kraft, and Lorelei A. Mucci. "Sniffing Out Significant 'Pee Values': Genome-Wide Association Study of Asparagus Anosmia," *British Medical Journal*, December 13, 2016, 355.

On vajacials:
Chan, Mi-Anne, "I Got a Facial on My Vagina—& Loved Every Minute of It." *Refinery29*, April 17, 2017.
Chung, Madelyn, "What Happened When I Got a Vajacial—a Facial for My Vagina," Huffington Post Canada, February 9, 2015.
Hsieh, Carina, "6 Things to Know About Getting a Vajacial [NSFW]," *Cosmopolitan*, September 6, 2017.

Statistics on ER visits due to pubic grooming accidents:
Glass, Allison S., Herman S. Bagga, Gregory E. Tasian, Patrick B. Fisher, Charles E. McCulloch, Sarah D. Blaschko, Jack W. McAninch, and Benjamin N. Breyer, "Pubic Hair Grooming Injuries Presenting to U.S. Emergency Departments," *Urology* 80(6), December 2012, 1187–91.

Products mentioned:
Betty Beauty, www.bettybeauty.com.
miniKINI, www.minikinicolour.com.

PRINCIPLE #3: THE SECRET TO BOOSTING YOUR LIBIDO ISN'T USUALLY IN A PRESCRIPTION BOTTLE

General background on women's arousal:
Dahl, Ellen Støkken, and Nina Brochmann, *The Wonder Down Under: The Insider's Guide to the Anatomy, Biology, and Reality of the Vagina*, London: Quercus Books, 2018, 96–99.

On average frequency of sex:
Austin Institute for the Study of Family and Culture, Relationships in America survey, www.RelationshipsinAmerica.com.
Nuwer, Rachel, "The Enduring Enigma of Female Sexual Desire," BBC, July 1, 2016.

On asexuality:
Asexual Visibility and Education Network (AVEN), www.asexuality.org.
LGBT Proportion of Population: United States, UCLA School of Law Williams Insititute, williamsinstitute.law.ucla.edu/visualization/lgbt-stats/?topic=LGBT#density.
Miller, Anna Medaris, "Asexuality: The Invisible Orientation?" U.S. News & World Report, May 4, 2015, https://health.usnews.com/health-news/health-wellness/articles/2015/05 /04/asexuality-the-invisible-orientation.
Parente, Jeanderson Soares, and Grayce Alencar Albuquerque, "Asexuality: Dysfunction or

Sexual Orientation?," *Reproductive System & Sexual Disorders: Current Research* 5(3), July 27, 2016.

Parkin, Simon, "'I Have Never Felt Sexual Desire,'" BBC, June 22, 2016.

On women's brains during orgasm:

Firger, Jessica, "What Happens to Women's Brains When They Orgasm? Climaxing Doesn't Result in Neurological Switch Off," *Newsweek*, October 13, 2017.

Wise, Nan J., Eleni Frangos, and Barry R. Komisaruk, "Brain Activity Unique to Orgasm in Women: An fMRI Analysis," *Journal of Sexual Medicine* 14(11), November 2017, 1380–91.

On Viagra:

Bradford, Andrea, and Cindy Meston, "Correlates of Placebo Response in the Treatment of Sexual Dysfunction in Women: A Preliminary Report," *Journal of Sexual Medicine* 4(5), September 2007, 1345–51.

Stories of older women's sex lives:

Cloud, John, "The Science of Cougar Sex: Why Older Women Lust," *Time*, December 29, 2010.

Levin, Hallie, "5 Reasons Why Sex Is Better in Your 40s," Prevention, June 19, 2015.

Statistics on low sex drive over lifetime:

Zeleke, Berihun M., Robin J. Bell, Baki Billah, and Susan R. Davis, "Hypoactive Sexual Desire Dysfunction in Community-Dwelling Older Women," *Menopause* 24(4), April 2017, 391–99.

Nuwer, Rachel, "The Enduring Enigma of Female Sexual Desire," BBC, July 1, 2016.

Mitchell, Kirstin R., Catherine H. Mercer, George B. Ploubidis, Kyle G. Jones, Jessica Datta, Nigel Field, Andrew J. Copas, Clare Tanton, Bob Erens, Pam Sonnenberg, Soazig Clifton, Wendy Macdowall, Andrew Phelps, Anne M. Johnson, and Kaye Wellings, "Sexual Function in Britain: Findings from the Third National Survey of Sexual Attitudes and Lifestyles," *Lancet* 382(9907), November 30–December 6, 2013, 1817–29.

On medical problems related to libido:

"FAQs: Your Sexual Health," American College of Obstetricians and Gynecologists, www .acog.org/Patients/FAQs/Your-Sexual-Health.

"National Diabetes Statistics Report, 2017: Estimates of Diabetes and Its Burden in the United States," American Diabetes Association, www.diabetes.org/assets/pdfs/basics /cdc-statistics-report-2017.pdf.

American Heart Association, www.heart.org.

"Sexual Difficulties in Women," American Sexual Health Association, www.ashasexualhealth.org/sexual-health/womens-health/sexual-difficulties.

"Sexual Dysfunction and Disease," Cleveland Clinic, my.clevelandclinic.org/health/diseases
/9125-sexual-dysfunction-and-disease.
"How Does Rheumatoid Arthritis Affect Sexual Function?" International Society for Sexual
Medicine, www.issm.info/sexual-health-qa/how-does-rheumatoid-arthritis-affect-sexual
-function.
"Matters of the Heart: Sex and Cardiovascular Disease," Harvard Health Publishing,
www.health.harvard.edu.
"Low Sex Drive in Women," Mayo Clinic, www.mayoclinic.org/diseases-conditions/low-sex
-drive-in-women/diagnosis-treatment/drc-20374561.
"Medications That Can Affect Sexual Desire and Pleasure," Our Bodies, Ourselves,
www.ourbodiesourselves.org/book-excerpts/health-article/medications-affecting-sexual
-desire-pleasure.
U.S. Department of Health & Human Services, www.womenshealth.gov.
U.S. National Library of Medicine, medlineplus.gov/thyroiddiseases.html.
Nascimiento, Elisabete Rodrigues, Ana Claudia Ornelas Maia, Valeska Pereira, Gastao
Soares-Fiho, Antonio Egidio Nardi, and Adriana Cardoso Silva, "Sexual Dysfunc-
tion and Cardiovascular Diseases: A Systematic Review of Prevalence," *Clinics* 68(11),
November 2013, 1462–68.
O'Connor, Amy, "Decreased Sex Drive During Pregnancy," What to Expect, June 1,
2018.

On low libido due to birth control pills:
Pastor, Zlatko, Katerina Holla, and Roman Chmel, "The Influence of Combined Oral
Contraceptives on Female Sexual Desire: A Systematic Review," *European Journal of
Contraception & Reproductive Health Care* 18(1), February 2013, 27–43.

Types of sexual dysfunction in women:
IsHak, Waguih William, and Gabriel Tobia, "DSM-5 Changes in Diagnostic Criteria of
Sexual Dysfunctions," *Reproductive System and Reproductive Sexual Disorders: Current
Research* 2(2), 2013.

PRINCIPLE #4: DISCOVER WHO YOU ARE IN BED—EVERY DAY

Background on Queen V superpowers:
"How to Be Multi-Orgasmic," Everyday Health, www.everydayhealth.com/sexual-health
/how-multi-gasmic.
"What Is 'Edging' and Why Might It Be Employed?" International Society for Sexual
Medicine, www.issm.info/sexual-health-qa/what-is-edging-and-why-might-it-be
-employed.
Cacciari, Licia Pazzoto, Anice Campos Pássaro, Amanda C. Amorim, and Isabel C. N.
Sacco, "High Spatial Resolution Pressure Distribution of the Vaginal Canal in Pompoir

Practitioners: A Biomechanical Approach for Assessing the Pelvic Floor," *Clinical Bio-mechanics* 47, August 2017, 53–60.

Denise Da Costa, pelvic floor expert, www.pompoirbook.com.

Salama, Samuel, Florence Boitrelle, Amélie Gauquelin, Lydia Malagrida, Nicolas Thiounn, and Pierre Desvaux, "Nature and Origin of 'Squirting' in Female Sexuality," *Journal of Sexual Medicine* 12(3), March 2015, 661–66.

Streicher, Lauren, "Science Says Yes to Female Ejaculation," Everyday Health, August 25, 2016.

Weisman, Carrie, "The Ancient (and Largely Forgotten) Secret to Super-Orgasms," *Salon*, March 9, 2015.

On communication and body language:

Lapakko, David, "Communication Is 93% Nonverbal: An Urban Legend Proliferates," *Communication and Theater Association of Minnesota Journal* 34, 2007, 7–19.

Thompson, Jeff, "Is Nonverbal Communication a Numbers Game?," Psychology Today, September 30, 2011.

PRINCIPLE #5: GET AS DOWN AND DIRTY AS YOU WANT—BUT REMEMBER THIS

On sexy situations:

"Wax Play Beginners' Guide," Sex Talk About, December 24, 2018.

Brown, Joelle M., Kristen L. Hess, Stephen Brown, Colleen Murphy, Ava Lena Wald-man, and Marjan Hezareh, "Intravaginal Practices and Risk of Bacterial Vaginosis and Candidiasis Infection Among a Cohort of Women in the United States," *Obstetrics and Gynecology* 121(4), April 2013, 773–80.

Kassel, Gabrielle, "Whipped Cream, Baby Oil, and 6 Other Things You Should Never Use as Lube," Health, September 25, 2018.

"What's the Best Way to Clean Sex Toys?" BWell, www.brown.edu/campus-life/health/services/promotion/content/whats-best-way-clean-sex-toys.

Underhill, Allison, "The Essential Guide to Cleaning Your Sex Toys (Yes, There's a Right Way to Do It!)," Health.com, July 17, 2017.

Brennan, Faye, "5 Essential Tips for How to Clean Your Sex Toys," *Women's Health*, August 18, 2014.

National Survey of Sexual Health and Behavior (NSSHB), Indiana University Bloomington School of Public Health, www.nationalsexstudy.indiana.edu.

Herbenick, Debby, Michael Reece, Vanessa Schick, Stephanie Sanders, Brian Dodge, and J. Dennis Fortenberry, "An Event-Level Analysis of the Sexual Characteristics and Composition Among Adults Ages 18 to 59: Results from a National Probability Sample in the United States," *Journal of Sexual Medicine* 7 Suppl. 5(s5), October 2010, 346–61.

Chatel, Amanda, "Here's Your Complete Guide to Fingering a Woman," Bolde.

General background on infections:

American College of Obstetricians and Gynecologists, www.acog.org.

Centers for Disease Control and Prevention, www.cdc.gov/std/hpv/stats.htm.

Cleveland Clinic, my.clevelandclinic.org.

Mayo Clinic, www.mayoclinic.org.

Planned Parenthood, www.plannedparenthood.org.

U.S. National Library of Medicine, www.medlineplus.gov.

U.S. Department of Health & Human Services, www.hhs.gov.

Research on hepatitis C and fertility:

Karampatou, Aimilia, XueHan, Loreta A. Kondili, Gloria Taliani, Alessia Ciancio, Filo-
mena Morisco, Rosina Maria Critelli, Enrica Baraldi, Veronica Bernabucci, Giulia
Troshina, Maria Guarino, Simonetta Tagliavini, Federica D'Ambrosio, Laura Bristot,
Laura Turco, Stefano Rosato, Stefano Vella, Tommaso Trenti, Isabella Neri, Antonio
La Marca, Shivaji Manthena, Andrea S. Goldstein, Savino Bruno, Yanjun Bao, Yuri
Sanchez Gonzalez, and Erica Villa, "Premature Ovarian Senescence and a High Miscar-
riage Rate Impair Fertility in Women with HCV," *Journal of Hepatology* 68(1), Janu-
ary 2018, 33–41.

On the rise of gonorrhea:

"New CDC Analysis Shows Steep and Sustained Increases in STDs in Recent Years,"
Centers for Disease Control, www.cdc.gov/media/releases/2018/p0828-increases-in-stds
.html.

Recommendations on the HPV vaccine:

"HPV Vaccine Schedule and Dosing," Centers for Disease Control, www.cdc.gov/hpv/hcp
/schedules-recommendations.html.

On lubricants:

Adcox, Mariah, "How to Choose the Best Lube for Your Sex Life," Healthline.

Baum, Isadora, "Is It Safe to Use Coconut Oil as a Lube? Ob-Gyns Explain," Health,
May 28, 2019.

Nathman, Avital Norman, "The Truth About Organic Lubes," Vice, July 13, 2017.

PRINCIPLE #6: YOU NEED A PLATINUM-LEVEL PROTECTION PLAN—EVEN IF YOU'RE MARRIED

General background on birth control methods and effectiveness:

American College of Obstetricians and Gynecologists, www.acog.org.

Bedsider, an online birth control support network operated by Power to Decide, the cam-
paign to prevent unplanned pregnancy, www.bedsider.org.

Guttmacher Institute, www.guttmacher.org.

Harvard Health Publishing, www.health.harvard.edu.

Mayo Clinic, www.mayoclinic.org.
National Women's Health Network, www.nwhn.org/female-condoms.
Planned Parenthood, www.plannedparenthood.org.
U.S. Department of Health and Human Services, www.hhs.gov and womenshealth.gov.

Statistics about women's contraceptive methods:
"Contraceptive Use in the United States: July 2018 Fact Sheet," Guttmacher Institute,
    www.guttmacher.org/fact-sheet/contraceptive-use-united-states.
Bedsider, www.bedsider.org.

Statistics on condom usage:
Casey E. Copen, "Condom Use During Sexual Intercourse Among Women and Men Aged
    15–44 in the United States: 2011–2015 National Survey of Family Growth," Centers
    for Disease Control, National Health Statistics Report, August 10, 2017.

PRINCIPLE #7: ALWAYS PLAN YOUR
TRIP TO HIS NETHERLANDS

General background on male anatomy:
"Erection Ejaculation: How It Occurs," Cleveland Clinic, https://my.clevelandclinic.org
    /health/articles/10036-erection-ejaculation-how-it-occurs.
"What Are the Parts of the Male Sexual Anatomy?," Planned Parenthood,
    https://www.plannedparenthood.org/learn/health-and-wellness/sexual-and-reproductive
    -anatomy/what-are-parts-male-sexual-anatomy.

On circumcision:
Owings, Maria, Sayeedha Uddin, and Sonja Williams, "Trends in Circumcision for Male
    Newborns in U.S. Hospitals: 1979–2010," Centers for Disease Control, August 2013,
    www.cdc.gov/nchs/data/hestat/circumcision_2013/circumcision_2013.pdf.
"Circumcision (Male)," Mayo Clinic, https://www.mayoclinic.org/tests-procedures
    /circumcision/about/pac-20393550.
Morris, Brian J., Jake H. Waskett, Joya Banerjee, Richard G. Wamai, Aaron A.R. Tobian,
    Ronald H. Gray, Stefan A. Bailis, Robert C. Bailey, Jeffrey D. Klausner, Robin J. Will-
    court, Daniel T. Halperin, Thomas E Wiswell, and Adrian Mindel, "A 'Snip' in Time:
    What Is the Best Age to Circumcise?," *BMC Pediatrics* 12(20), February 28, 2012.
Purshotham Shenoy, Sunil, Prashanth Kallaje Marla, Pritham Sharma, Narayana Bhat,
    and Amrith Raj Rao, "Frenulum Sparing Circumcision: Step-by-Step Approach of a
    Novel Technique," *Journal of Clinical and Diagnostic Research* 9(12), December 2015,
    PC01–PC03.

On Peyronie's Disease:
"Peyronie's Disease," Mayo Clinic, https://www.mayoclinic.org/diseases-conditions
    /peyronies-disease/symptoms-causes/syc-20353468.

"Penile Curvature (Peyronie's Disease)," U.S. Department of Health and Human Services, https://www.niddk.nih.gov/health-information/urologic-diseases/penile-curvature-peyronies-disease.

Brody, Jane E., "A New Treatment for a Painful Penis Curvature," *New York Times*, February 11, 2019.

General background on sexually transmitted infections:
Centers for Disease Control, www.cdc.gov.
Mayo Clinic, www.mayoclinic.org.
Planned Parenthood, www.plannedparenthood.org.

On delayed testing for STIs:
Malek, Angela M., Chung-Chou H. Chang, Duncan B. Clark, and Robert L. Cook, "Delay in Seeking Care for Sexually Transmitted Diseases in Young Men and Women Attending a Public STD Clinic," *Open AIDS Journal* 7, June 14, 2013, 7–13.

Fode, Mikkel, Ferdinando Fusco, Larry Lipshultz, and Wolfgana Weidner, "Sexually Transmitted Disease and Male Infertility: A Systematic Review," *European Urology Focus* 2(4), October 2016, 383–93.

PRINCIPLE #8: KNOW WHEN TO LEAVE SEX TOYS TO THE PROFESSIONALS

General background on sex toys:
Kandi Burruss, www.bedroomkandi.com.
Angela Lieben, www.Liberator.com.

Additional product mentions:
Chakrubs, www.chakrubs.com.
Njoy, www.njoytoys.com.
Organic Loven, www.organicloven.com.

PRINCIPLE #9: TREAT YOUR PERIOD LIKE A FRENEMY

On menstruation, first moon parties, and cycle syncing:
"FAQs: Your First Period (Especially for Teens)," American College of Obstetricians and Gynecologists, https://www.acog.org/Patients/FAQs/Your-First-Period-Especially-for-Teens.

"Menstrual Cycle: What's Normal, What's Not," Mayo Clinic, https://www.mayoclinic.org/healthy-lifestyle/womens-health/in-depth/menstrual-cycle/art-20047186.

Devine, Lucy, "Parents Are Throwing Their Daughters Period Parties," *New York Post*, July 16, 2018.

Fisher, Claudia, "Why You Should Throw Your Daughter a 'First-Period' Party," *Real Simple*, July 12, 2018.

Rettner, Rachael, "Women's Periods Don't Really Sync Up When They Live Together," Live
    Science, April 13, 2017.
Watson, Kathryn, author; Weatherspoon, Deborah, medical reviewer, "Period Syncing: Real
    Phenomenon or Popular Myth?," Healthline, January 23, 2019.

On IUDs and menstruation:
"Will an IUD Make Your Period Go Away?," Bedsider, https://www.bedsider.org/features
    /937-will-an-iud-make-your-period-go-away.
"Mirena (Hormonal IUD)," Mayo Clinic, https://www.mayoclinic.org/tests-procedures
    /mirena/about/pac-20391354.

On menstrual cycle phases:
Knudtson, Jennifer, and Jessica E. McLaughlin, "Menstrual Cycle," Merck Manuals,
    https://www.merckmanuals.com/home/women-s-health-issues/biology-of-the-female
    -reproductive-system/menstrual-cycle.
"Stages of the Menstrual Cycle," Healthline, www.healthline.com/health/womens-health
    /stages-of-menstrual-cycle.
"Mittelschmerz," Mayo Clinic, https://www.mayoclinic.org/diseases-conditions
    /mittelschmerz/symptoms-causes/syc-20375122.
"Charting Your Menstrual Cycle," Our Bodies, Ourselves, April 1, 2014, https://www
    .ourbodiesourselves.org/book-excerpts/health-article/charting-your-menstrual-cycle.
Reed, Beverly G., and Bruce R. Carr, "The Normal Menstrual Cycle and the Control of
    Ovulation," in K. R. Feingold, B. Anawalt, A. Boyce, et al., eds., *Endotext*, South Dart-
    mouth, MA: MDText.com, August 5, 2018.

Statistics on PMDD:
"PMDD/PMS," MGH Center for Women's Mental Health, www.womensmentalhealth.org
    /specialty-clinics/pms-and-pmdd.

General background on period problems:
American College of Obstetricians and Gynecologists, www.acog.org.
American Migraine Foundation, www.americanmigrainefoundation.org.
Centers for Disease Control, www.cdc.org.
Cleveland Clinic, my.clevelandclinic.org.
Johns Hopkins Medicine, www.hopkinsmedicine.org.
Mayo Clinic, www.mayoclinic.org.
U.S. Department of Health & Human Services, ods.od.nih.gov.

On natural remedies for dysmenorrhea:
Barnard, Neal D., A. R. Scialli, Donna Hurlock, and Patricia Bertron, "Diet and
    Sex-Hormone Binding Globulin, Dysmenorrhea, and Premenstrual Symptoms,"
    Obstetrics and Gynecology 95(2), February 2000, 245–50.
Hosseinlou, Abdollah, V. Alinejad, M. Mahdi Alinejad, and Nader Aghakhani, "The Effects
    of Fish Oil Capsules and Vitamin B1 Tablets on Duration and Severity of Dysmenor-
    rhea in Students of High School in Urmia-Iran," *Global Journal of Health Science* 6(7),
    September 18, 2014, 124–29.

Ou, Ming-Chiu, Tsung-Fu Hsu, Andrew C. Lai, Yu-Ting Lin, and Chia-Ching Lin, "Pain Relief Assessment by Aromatic Essential Oil Massage on Outpatients with Primary Dysmenorrhea: A Randomized, Double-Blind Clinical Trial," *Journal of Obstetrics and Gynaecology Research* 38(5), May 2012, 817–22.

Smith, C. A., X. Zhu, L. He, and J. Song, "Acupuncture for Primary Dysmenorrhoea," *Cochrane Database of Systematic Reviews* 1, January 19, 2011.

Vaziri, Farideh, Azam Hoseini, Farahnaz Kamali, Khadijeh kh k Abdali, Mohamadjavad Hadianfard, and Mehrab Sayadi, "Comparing the Effects of Aerobic and Stretching Exercises on the Intensity of Primary Dysmenorrhea in the Students of Universities of Bushehr," *Journal of Family and Reproductive Health* 9(1), 23–28.

Statistics on dysmenorrhea:

Latthe, Pallavi, Rita Champaneria, and Khalid Khan, "Dysmenorrhea," *American Family Physician* 85(4), February 15, 2012, 386–87, www.aafp.org/afp/2012/0215/p386 .html.

Grandi, Giovanni, Serena Ferrari, Anjeza Xholli, Marianna Cannoletta, Federica Palma, Cecilia Romani, Annibale Volpe, and Angelo Cagnacci, "Prevalence of Menstrual Pain in Young Women: What Is Dysmenorrhea?" *Journal of Pain Research* 5, June 2012, 169–74.

Statistics on tampon usage:

Fetters, Ashley, "The Tampon: A History," *Atlantic*, June 1, 2015.

Woeller, Kara E., Kenneth W. Miller, Amy L. Robertson-Smith, and Lisa C. Bohman, "Impact of Advertising on Tampon Wear-Time Practices," *Clinical Medicine Insights* 8, November 29, 2015, 29–38.

General background on menopause:

"Diet Might Delay—or Hasten—the Onset of Menopause," Harvard Health Publishing, August 2018, www.health.harvard.edu/womens-health/diet-might-delay-or-hasten-the -onset-of-menopause.

"Menopause," Mayo Clinic, www.mayoclinic.org/diseases-conditions/menopause/symptoms -causes/syc-20353397.

"What Is Menopause?," National Institute on Aging, www.nia.nih.gov/health/what -menopause.

Sapre, Shilpa, and Ratna Thakur, "Lifestyle and Dietary Factors Determine Age at Natural Menopause," *Journal of Mid-Life Health* 5(1), January–March 2014, 3–5.

PRINCIPLE #10: KNOW YOUR BREASTS LIKE YOU KNOW YOUR WAY HOME

On breasts and breast cancer:

"Mucinous (Colloid) Breast Cancer," Johns Hopkins Medicine, Breast Cancer Program, www.hopkinsmedicine.org/kimmel_cancer_center/centers/breast_cancer_program /treatment_and_services/rare_breast_tumors/mucinous_breast_cancer.html.

"U.S. Breast Cancer Statistics," Breastcancer.org, www.breastcancer.org/symptoms /understand_bc/statistics.

"Types of Breast Cancer," American Cancer Society, www.cancer.org/cancer/breast-cancer /understanding-a-breast-cancer-diagnosis/types-of-breast-cancer.html.

"What Is Breast Cancer?," Centers for Disease Control, www.cdc.gov/cancer/breast/basic _info/what-is-breast-cancer.htm.

"Fibrocystic Breasts," Mayo Clinic, www.mayoclinic.org/diseases-conditions/fibrocystic -breasts/symptoms-causes/syc-20350438.

"Anatomy of the Breast," Memorial Sloan Kettering Cancer Center, www.mskcc.org/cancer -care/types/breast/anatomy-breast.

"Breast Cancer Fact Sheet," Susan G. Komen, August 2018, ww5.komen.org/uploadedFiles /_Komen/Content/About_Us/Media_Center/Newsroom/breast-cancer-fact-sheet -august-2018.pdf.

"Breast Self-Exam," U.S. National Library of Medicine, https://medlineplus.gov/ency/article /001993.htm.

On fibrocystic breasts:

Cerrato, Felecia, and Brian I. Labow, "Diagnosis and Management of Fibroadenomas in the Adolescent Breast," *Seminars in Plastic Surgery* 27(1), February 2013, 23–25.

Lee, Michelle, and Hooman T. Soltanian, "Breast Fibroadenomas in Adolescents: Current Perspectives," *Adolescent Health, Medicine and Therapeutics* 6, September 2015, 159–63.

Santen, Richard J., "Benign Breast Disease in Women," in K. R. Feingold, B. Anawalt, A. Boyce, et al., eds., *Endotext*, South Dartmouth, MA: MDText.com, May 25, 2018.

"Fibrocystic Breasts," Mayo Clinic, www.mayoclinic.org/diseases-conditions/fibrocystic -breasts/diagnosis-treatment/drc-20350442.

"Benign Breast Conditions," Susan G. Komen, ww5.komen.org/BreastCancer /BenignConditions.html.

Statistics on the number of cells in the human body:

Sender, Ron, Shai Fuchs, and Ron Milo, "Revised Estimates for the Number of Human and Bacteria Cells in the Body," *PLoS Biology* 14(8), August 19, 2016.

On bra size survey:

Talarico, Brittany, "Even Victoria's Secret Models Aren't Wearing the Right Bra Size: Tips and Tricks from the Experts," *People*, August 14, 2018.

On how to do a breast self-exam:

"Breast Self-Exam," BreastCancer.org, www.breastcancer.org/symptoms/testing/types/self _exam.

"Breast Self-Exam for Breast Awareness," Mayo Clinic, www.mayoclinic.org/tests -procedures/breast-exam/about/pac-20393237.

"Breast Self-Exam," U.S. National Library of Medicine, www.medlineplus.gov/ency/article /001993.htm.

On breast changes and recommended exams:

"Factors That Affect Risk: Age," Susan G. Komen, ww5.komen.org/BreastCancer
/GettingOlder.html.

Statistics on genetics and breast cancer:

Haber, Gillian, Nasar U. Ahmed, and Vukosava Pekovic, "Family History of Cancer and Its
Association with Breast Cancer Risk Perception and Repeat Mammography," *American
Journal of Public Health* 102(12), October 2012, 2322–29.

Statistics on breast cancer five-year survival rate:

"Study Estimates Number of U.S. Women Living with Metastatic Breast Cancer," National
Cancer Institute, May 18, 2017, www.cancer.gov/news-events/press-releases/2017
/metastatic-breast-cancer-survival-rates.

"Metastatic Breast Cancer," Susan G. Komen, ww5.komen.org/BreastCancer/Metastatic
BreastCancerIntroduction.html.

"Survival Rates for Breast Cancer," American Cancer Society, www.cancer.org/cancer/breast
-cancer/understanding-a-breast-cancer-diagnosis/breast-cancer-survival-rates.html.

On lives saved due to mammography and treatment advances:

Hendrick, R. Edward, Jay A. Baker, and Mark A. Helvie, "Breast Cancer Deaths Averted
Over 3 Decades," *Cancer* 125(9), May 1, 2019, 1482–88.

PRINCIPLE #11: IF YOU DON'T CONTROL YOUR FERTILITY, IT WILL CONTROL YOU

General background on female anatomy:

American Pregnancy Association, americanpregnancy.org.

"Female Reproductive System," Cleveland Clinic, my.clevelandclinic.org/health/articles
/9118-female-reproductive-system.

"Human Body: Uterine Tube (Fallopian Tube)," Healthline, www.healthline.com/human
-body-maps/fallopian-tubes#1.

"Internal Organs: Uterus, Fallopian Tubes, Ovaries," Our Bodies, Ourselves,
www.ourbodiesourselves.org/book-excerpts/health-article/internal-organs-uterus
-fallopian-tubes-ovaries.

"Ectopic Pregnancy," Planned Parenthood, https://www.plannedparenthood.org/learn
/pregnancy/ectopic-pregnancy.

Statistics about number of eggs:

"Female Reproductive System," Cleveland Clinic, my.clevelandclinic.org/health/articles
/9118-female-reproductive-system.

On genetic defects and infertility:

"FAQs: Evaluating Infertility," American College of Obstetricians and Gynecologists, www
.acog.org/Patients/FAQs/Evaluating-Infertility.

"Treatments & Conditions: Uterine Anomaly," Columbia University Irving Medical Center, www.columbiadoctors.org/condition/uterine-anomaly.

"Septate Uterus," Healthline, www.healthline.com/health/septate-uterus.

"A–Z Health Topics: Infertility," U.S. Department of Health & Human Services, Office on Women's Health, www.womenshealth.gov/a-z-topics/infertility.

Zorrilla, Michelle, and Alexander N. Yatsenko, "The Genetics of Infertility: Current Status of the Field," *Current Genetic Medicine Reports* 1(4), October 16, 2013.

Statistics about male factor infertility:

Kumar, Naina, and Amit K. Singh, "Trends of Male Factor Infertility, an Important Cause of Infertility: A Review of Literature," *Journal of Human Reproductive Sciences* 8(4), January 2016, 191–96.

Resources on fertility treatments:

American Pregnancy Association, www.americanpregnancy.org.

Centers for Disease Control, www.cdc.gov.

Child Welfare Information Gateway, www.childwelfare.gov.

Mayo Clinic, www.mayoclinic.org.

Resolve, the National Infertility Association, www.resolve.org.

"About Surrogacy," Surrogate.com, www.surrogate.com/about-surrogacy/types-of-surrogacy/types-of-surrogacy.

General background on medical and surgical abortion:

American Pregnancy Association, www.americanpregnancy.org.

Planned Parenthood, www.plannedparenthood.org.

Statistics on teen pregnancy:

"About Teen Pregnancy," Centers for Disease Control, www.cdc.gov/teenpregnancy/about/index.htm.

"Decrease in Teen Pregnancy," U.S. Department of Health & Human Services, Office on Women's Health, www.womenshealth.gov/30-achievements/09.

Statistics on abortions:

"Abortion Is a Common Experience for U.S. Women, Despite Dramatic Declines in Rates," Guttmacher Institute, October 19, 2017, www.guttmacher.org/news-release/2017/abortion-common-experience-us-women-despite-dramatic-declines-rates.

PRINCIPLE #12: STOP WITH THE DÉJÀ VU APPOINTMENTS

General background on fibroids:

American College of Obstetrics and Gynecology, www.acog.org.

Mayo Clinic, www.mayoclinic.org.

UCLA Health, obgyn.ucla.edu/fibroids.

U.S. Department of Health & Human Services, Office on Women's Health, www.womenshealth.gov.

On adenomyosis and endometriosis:

"About Endometriosis," National Institutes of Health, www.nichd.nih.gov/health/topics /endometri/conditioninfo.

"Fibroid-like Conditions: Adenomyosis and Endometrial Polyps," Brigham Health, Brigham and Women's Hospital, https://www.brighamandwomens.org/obgyn /infertility-reproductive-surgery/cysts-and-fibroids/fibroid-line-conditions-adenomyosis -and-endometrial-polyps.

Kilpatrick, Charlie C., "Uterine Adenomyosis," Merck Manuals, www.merckmanuals .com/professional/gynecology-and-obstetrics/benign-gynecologic-lesions/uterine -adenomyosis.

Mayo Clinic, www.mayoclinic.org.

U.S. Department of Health & Human Services, Office on Women's Health, www.womenshealth.gov.

On dyspareunia:

"Dyspareunia—When Sex Hurts," American Sexual Health Association, www.ashasexualhealth.org/dyspareunia-sex-hurts.

On pelvic organ prolapse:

"FAQs: Surgery for Pelvic Organ Prolapse," American College of Obstetrics and Gynecology, www.acog.org/Patients/FAQs/Surgery-for-Pelvic-Organ-Prolapse.

"Pelvic Organ Prolapse," U.S. Department of Health & Human Services, Office on Women's Health, www.womenshealth.gov/files/documents/fact-sheet-pelvic-organ -prolapse.pdf.

On urge incontinence:

"Urge Incontinence," U.S. National Library of Medicine, medlineplus.gov/ency/article /001270.htm.

"Urinary Incontinence in Women," Johns Hopkins Medicine, www.hopkinsmedicine.org /health/conditions-and-diseases/urinary-incontinence/urinary-incontinence-in-women.

ACKNOWLEDGMENTS

It takes a village to raise a child—and it has taken a whole kingdom to create *The Queen V.* So I want to thank each and every person who had a hand in helping me bring this book to life.

First and foremost are my patients, because there wouldn't be a book without you. I've been writing *The Queen V* in my head since day one of my residency at the Medical Center of Central Georgia. I'll never forget when a patient started telling me about her "history correction" (meaning her "hysterectomy"). I jotted that story down on a piece of paper and it was the first of many. I remember thinking that it wasn't just me or women from my home state of Mississippi who need to know more about women's health. It wasn't just women in Georgia. It was all of us. And I was going to take on the charge.

Thanks to the Braxton sisters, I was blessed to meet Vincent Herbert, who knew that when you have big dreams (like I did) you need big representation. He connected me to Santini Reali, Cait Hoyt, and everyone at Creative Artists Agency who I'm ever grateful to for helping turn those big dreams into an incredible reality.

Thanks to Purveyor of Pops, Bravo TV, and *Married to Medicine.* Without Purveyor of Pops (Matt Anderson and Nate Green), Bravo TV (Toni Tonge, I will never forget that driver you hooked me up with), and the tireless production crew and must-see-TV cast of *Married to Medicine*, I wouldn't have Andy Cohen in my life.

My gratitude goes out to Andy Cohen, who heard and believed in my vision to educate, uplift, and inspire Queen Vs all over the world. I wouldn't be at this place and time in my life had Andy not been enthralled by the stories I have to tell. When I told him about my idea for this book, he helped turn it into the pages you're reading right now. I'm so very deeply honored to have written one of the first books in his imprint.

Libby Burton and Gillian Blake at Henry Holt have my eternal gratitude for shepherding this book from start to finish with incredible insight
and thoughtfulness.

I want to thank Lynya Floyd, my collaborator, whom I picked from
a long list of options because of her decades of work as a health journal-
ist, her resourcefulness, and her similar passion for uplifting women. I'm
also grateful for illustrator Adeola Ajayi (my adoptive son) and his artistic
hand, who crafted the vaginal flowers you see in the book.

I'm not quite sure how I'd make it through each day without my coor-
dinator/assistant/confidant Eboni Cummings. Every woman should be as
lucky as I am to have someone who never tires of me bouncing ideas off
her, who is honest with me when I'm crazy, who can fight with me like a
sibling, and still shows me love and respect. Eboni, Nybria Baker, Petrina
Forts, Tiffany White, and Dr. Rachel Paccione all devoted time to reading
drafts of this book and giving me brilliant insights into what they loved
and what had to go. I so appreciate you ladies for that!

Whenever I didn't know enough about a topic, I found the go-to expert
in the field to talk about it. So many health advocates were kind enough to
share their knowledge for this book, including John R. Miklos, MD; Jennifer
Hunt, PT, DPT; Tiffanie Davis Henry, PhD; Tasneem "Dr. Taz" Bhatia,
MD; Angela Lieben; Jennifer L. Amerson, MD; Ginny Ehrlich, D.Ed,
MPH, MS; Jamila Perritt, MD, MPH; and Desireé McCarthy-Keith, MD.

It's not easy on a spouse when you work long days at a hospital and
have long days of filming a television show, followed by nights of typing
away on a laptop. My husband, Curtis Berry, was not only tolerant of my
time and commitment to this project but was also a great sounding board.
Thank you for being a great listener.

No matter how grown you are, you always have to thank your parents. After all, it was my momma who sparked my passion for women's
health when I was a child, and my father who I get so much of my sense
of humor from (I just don't cuss like he did). Thank you to the listening ears of my sister, Kasandra Bailey, and her daughters, Summer and
Kandice, who are both studying to be physicians like me. They are my
cheerleaders.

Thank you to my BFFs Annie, Courtney, LaKesha, Terrinee, and Sidney; you are my greatest encouragers.

Thank you to my glam squad Joyua Gibson, Rhondalyn Patterson, and Messiah Marcial, photographer Robert Ector, and stylist Tesa Render, who fulfilled the vision for *The Queen V*'s cover with their creativity and tenacity.

Finally, I want to praise God, who has given me the ability to have peace that surpasses all understanding in all situations. His peace allows me to use my life to inspire, encourage, educate, and uplift others—especially women.

INDEX

deep vein thrombosis (DVT), 116
déjà vu conditions, 220–35
  common, 224–31
dental dam, 66, 83, 84, 86, 124
deodorant, 28
depilatory cream, 34
Depo-Provera, 114
depression, 59, 61, 157, 158
designer vaginas, 19–24
diabetes, 60, 93, 198, 203
diaphragm, 110–11, 165
dildos, 67, 141, 146, 147
discharge, 2, 12, 29–30, 90, 139
  bacterial vaginosis, 93–94
  chlamydia, 96, 104
  forgotten tampon, 166
  gonorrhea, 97, 135, 137
  normal, 29–30
  trichomoniasis, 99, 116
  yeast infection, 92–93
divorce, 48, 202
doctors, 91, 93, 126, 158, 175, 182,
  232–33
  abortion, 217–18
  annual exam, 90
  as patients, 171
  breast cancer, 192
  choice of surgeon, 22–23
  déjà vu appointments, 220–25
  fertility, 197, 198, 211–13
  prep for appointment, 17–18,
  234–35
  See also gynecologist
douching, 28, 30–31, 94, 166
dryness, vaginal, 29, 60–61, 199,
  229
dysmenorrhea, 159–60
dyspareunia, 228–30

edging, 69
eggs, 156, 196, 197, 200
  donor, 206, 214
  fertilized, 199, 200, 205, 206
  freezing, 203, 204, 212–14
  infertility and, 196–98, 200, 205–7,
  212–14
Ehrlich, Ginny, 208–11
emergency contraceptives (EC),
  119–20
endometrial ablation, 154

endometriosis, 153, 159, 201, 205, 226–28
  treatment, 227
erotica, 67–68
estrogen, 47, 182, 199
  birth control, 113, 114, 116, 159
  menopause and, 61, 167, 178
  menstrual cycle and, 155, 158
exercise, xxxi, 160, 186, 188
  pelvic, 38–41

fallopian tubes, 156, 199–200, 203, 212
fantasy, 223–24
fear, 223
  breast cancer and, 180, 191, 192
feet, 67
  toeing and footplay, 86
female condom, 104, 109–10
fertility, 92, 195–219, 223
  abortion and, 207–8, 214–18
  advice, 211–14
  anatomy and, 199–200
  birth control and, 204, 208–11
  cancer and, 213–14
  causes of infertility, 200–202
  control of, 202–4
  definition of infertility, 198
  drugs, 196, 197
  miscarriage, 195–96, 198, 201
  problems, 92, 99, 100, 133, 195–219,
  226, 227
  teenage, 208–11
  treatments, 204, 205–7
fertility awareness methods (FAMs),
  111, 205
fibroids, 159, 160, 201, 203, 220, 221,
  223, 225–26
  treatment, 223, 224, 226
finances, 52–53, 185–86, 197, 222–23
  abortion and, 217
  breast cancer and, 185–86, 189
  fertility treatments, 206–7
fingering, 87
fisting, 87
follicular phase, 155
folliculitis, 13–14
food, 29, 41, 140, 158, 167, 168, 196, 224
  breast cancer and, 186–88
  effects on vagina, 29
  healthy, 186–88
  in vagina, 140

jade eggs, 39
jock itch, 86
journaling, 185

Kegels, 38, 39
kidneys, 94, 95
kissing, 97, 126

labia, 4–12, 142
  anatomy, 4–11
  bleaching, 37
  lumps and bumps, 13–18, 90
  majora, 4–12, 19, 22
  minora, 4–12, 19, 20, 21
  surgery, 19–24
labiaplasty, 19, 21, 22, 23
laser treatments, 35
laziness, 75
lesbians, 116–17, 141, 205
libido, 43–63, 156, 199
  age and, 46–47
  bad sex and, 50–51
  Four S's, 51–55
  Intentional Loving and, 54–55
  low, 44–51, 56–63
  medical problems and, 59–61
  myths about, 44–47
  science of, 43–44
  supplements, 62–63
  therapy and, 56–58, 73–77
  types of sexual dysfunction in women, 61–62
  Vaginal Personality and, 48–49
Lieben, Angela, 146–48
liver, and hepatitis, 98–99
lotions, 80–81
lubricants, 5, 80–82, 84, 87, 101–3, 141
  all-natural, 102–3
  anal sex, 85–86
  hybrid, 102
  oil-based, 102
  protection of vagina, 80–81, 101–3
  silicone-based, 102
  sperm-friendly, 84
  water-based, 102
lumpectomy, 171, 192
lumps and bumps, 13–18, 90, 128, 132, 137
  answers for your doctor, 17–18

cysts, 14–15
folliculitis, 13–14
fordyce spots, 14
genital herpes, 16
genital warts, 15–16
melanomas, 16–17
skin tags, 15, 20
luteal phase, 156

magnesium, 158
mammograms, 172, 179, 189–91, 195
marriage, 48, 74, 107, 121, 233
  fertility problems, 197–98, 201–2
  Four S's and, 51–55
  honeymoon cystitis, 85, 95
  infidelity, 121–26
  libido issues, 43–63
  protection plans, 121–26
  STI testing, 121
Mary Jane, xix, xxviii–xxix, 1–2, 19, 48, 66, 104, 139, 145
mastectomy, 172, 192
masturbation, 25, 50, 79
  low sex drive and, 50
McCarthy-Keith, Desireé, 211–14
medical history, 116, 167, 178, 179
medications, 46, 47, 159, 161
  abortion, 119, 207, 215
  for common infections, 92–103
  libido and, 59–60, 62
  for migraines, 158–59
meditation, xxxi
melanomas, 16–17
menopause, 60–61, 141, 154, 166–69, 178, 196, 199, 229
  managing, 166–69
  perimenopause, 117, 166, 178
menstrual cup, 164, 165
menstrual cycle, phases of, 155–56
migraines, 117, 158–59
Miklos, John R., 21–24
miscarriage, 195–96, 198, 201, 207
moles, 16–17
monogamy, 121, 138
mons pubis, 4, 5, 13
MRI, 172, 179, 227, 228
myomectomy, 226

ABOUT THE AUTHOR

JACKIE WALTERS, known to hundreds of thousands of fans as "Dr. Jackie," has been a practicing OB-GYN since 1997. A two-time breast cancer survivor, she is the founder of the 50 Shades of Pink Foundation, an organization established in 2013 to treat the inner and outer beauty of survivors. One of the stars of Bravo's hit reality series *Married to Medicine*, she has also been featured on HLN and in *Essence*, *Glamour*, *People*, Rolling Out, and the *Atlanta Journal-Constitution*. She lives in Atlanta.